THE TRUTH ABOUT AIDS

Many useful facts and opinions about the medical and social aspects of AIDS.

Nursing Times

Should be available to every GP for his own use and for lending to those concerned ... well referenced yet written with a minimum of technical jargon.

The Physician

A wealth of research and published material from medical and popular sources in a detailed and extensively referenced book.

British Medical Journal

Useful and interesting book that patients will read and benefit from.

Journal of Royal College of General Practitioners

Excellent and thoroughly readable book.

Caring Professions Concern

Probably the best single volume of the whole AIDS issue available today. I recommend it to pastors and those with care responsibility as well as others with more general interest.

Restoration

If *Which?* offers a best buy then *The Truth About AIDS* is my choice ... the tone, suggestions and response seem to mirror exactly what Jesus would require of us all in the current crisis.

Third Way

Personal faith, questions and weaknesses are honestly shared by a Christian doctor who does not regard the finality of death as failure.

Life and Work

Dr Patrick Dixon *(MA, Cambridge University; MB BS, London University) trained at King's College Cambridge, Charing Cross Hospital London, and St Joseph's Hospice in Hackney. He was part of a Terminal Care Team, advising on the care of people dying in hospitals and at home. Dr Dixon is director of AIDS Care Education and Training (ACET) which is a church-based organisation providing a nationwide network of practical volunteer and professional help to people with AIDS at home. ACET also provides schools with AIDS education. The home care networks are supervised by hospice-style medical teams. ACET is also actively supporting overseas projects.*

Dr Dixon has lived in Africa and the United States and has revisited both to see firsthand the United States and African AIDS disasters. He is married with four children, and lives in a family-based community with four others. He is one of the elders of Ealing Christian Fellowship and a member of the Pioneer Trust.

The Truth About AIDS

DR PATRICK DIXON

KINGSWAY PUBLICATIONS
EASTBOURNE

First published 1987
Reprinted 1988
This revised edition 1990

British Library Cataloguing in Publication Data

Dixon, Patrick
The truth about AIDS. – 2nd ed.
1. Man. AIDS
I. Title
616.9792

ISBN 0–86065–880–5

Printed in Great Britain for
KINGSWAY PUBLICATIONS LTD
1 St Anne's Road, Eastbourne, E Sussex BN21 3UN by
Courier International Ltd, Tiptree, Essex.
Typeset by Watermark, Cromer, Norfolk

To all who feel rejected because of AIDS

Contents

Abbreviations

I hate jargon.

If you want a book full of technical terms then look elsewhere.

You will find a glossary at the back. It is not there to help you decipher this book, but to translate other things you may read or hear.

The terms 'body positive' or 'positive' are used throughout the book to describe where viral infection has taken place and the blood test is positive, although the person may be completely well.

The term 'HIV' is used to describe a group of viruses which cause AIDS or AIDS-like syndromes in some or all of those infected. Doctors love to give things long names such as 'human T-lymphotropic virus type III', which is so long no one can be bothered to use it. It then becomes known as HTLV-III or HIV.

'AIDS' is the only other abbreviation used often. It is short for Acquired Immune Deficiency Syndrome. I use it only because it is now widely accepted.

Many people who have developed AIDS, their families, and their friends dislike the implied meanings of phrases such as AIDS sufferer, AIDS patient, and AIDS victim. They prefer 'people who have developed AIDS'. I have tried to respect that but to substitute five words for two throughout the book became cumbersome.

The message of this book is that AIDS is not just a medical condition. AIDS represents a lot of individual people who are experiencing a devastating tragedy.

Often I have used he or his although the person could equally well be a woman. Please do not infer from this that AIDS is a male gay disease. As you will see, nothing could be further from the truth.

Preface to second edition

The first edition of this book in November 1987 caused quite a stir. Packed with the latest facts and figures on AIDS, and backed by literally hundreds of scientific references and footnotes, it challenged what was being said.

Written originally to motivate churches to get involved in a practical, caring response, it found a much wider audience. Since then several thousand new research papers have been published, governments have revised figures and forecasts, and major new problems have emerged. These are the reasons for a completely new edition.

Even in 1987 the African problem appeared vast, and Eastern Europe seemed likely to be hard hit. Both situations are more extensive than I feared then. Real progress on treatments and vaccines has been disappointingly slow despite press headlines. Western governments are revising down original forecasts for their own countries. This has led to abandonment of lower risk behaviour by some.

It is bizarre that now we are certain that at least 60% of all six million HIV infections worldwide has been heterosexually spread, some still say they do not accept significant heterosexual spread will happen in the West.

Stigma, rejection, social isolation, ignorance and fear are unfortunately still hugely present in many countries. People with AIDS continue to fight illness and die in appalling conditions, and in many countries a mixture of politics, culture and other sensitivities still prevent effective high-impact education campaigns.

As a direct result of this book, a major international church-based AIDS initiative was launched in the UK in June 1988, called ACET (AIDS Care Education and Training). ACET has since grown to become the largest independent provider of practical care to those ill with HIV/AIDS at home in the UK, and is also the UK's largest provider of face-to-face AIDS lessons in schools. ACET is also working overseas in partnership with churches, together with government and other non-governmental organisations. ACET has ongoing work in Uganda and Romania, with planned involvement also in Zimbabwe, Tanzania, Poland, Australia and New Zealand. The need has never been more urgent for a practical, professionally-based response, backed by volunteers.

Whilst every country is unique, basic principles of unconditional care and high impact education remain the same. God calls us all, I believe, to accept all people and to extend his love to them regardless of whether or not we agree with what they do. My hope and prayer is that this new edition will further stimulate a massive, yet sensitive, worldwide response to AIDS.

August 1990

Preface to First Edition

To some people, it must seem an act of ultimate folly to write a book that becomes out-of-date a few months later. The lightning spread of HIV infection across the globe, the rate of change, the appearance of wonder cures and their hasty withdrawal after only a few months, are all things which make writers and publishers nervous. But this book had to be written. Every day I hear people who should know better make statements that are out-of-date and misleading.

This is a book written on the run: on aeroplanes, in airports, and on trains. It was written between speaking engagements, visiting dying patients, counselling their relatives, visiting San Francisco to see for myself the horror of that situation, and recently visiting Central Africa.

All the while research papers, reports, and press clippings poured in. In the last eighteen months, several thousand research papers have been published in American, German, Spanish, African, British, or other journals. A similar number of press articles and radio or television programmes have been made. I hope I have written a reasonable digest of all of them.

This book is about people. Details of names, places, times, and events have been altered where necessary to protect identity. If you think you are reading about someone or some place you know, you are probably mistaken. Some of the medical case reports in Chapter 3 are compiled from real events in a number of people's lives.

This book is written from the perspective of a doctor who is also a church leader.

Some Bible passages are written in the end notes. These need to be read in context. Almost any argument can be constructed out of isolated Bible quotations. For the last three years I have made it my business to read the Bible each year from start to finish—to catch its overall meaning and avoid 'verse grabbing' pitfalls. I encourage you to do the same.

Some parts of this book are sexually explicit and some may find this offensive. As a doctor I deal with real people in the real world who need accurate information and practical help. I regret giving offence but my goal is to save lives.

November 1987

Acknowledgements

Thank you firstly to Kingsway Publications who initially suggested that I write this book. Thank you to John Spencer FRCS who has been a continual source of wisdom and good counsel over the years and originally encouraged me when I was first thinking of becoming involved in the care of those who were very ill because of AIDS. He made many helpful suggestions to clarify parts of the manuscript that were ambiguous or obscure.

This book would not have been possible without the enormous practical care, support, and kindness from many in the church I belong to. A number of people made sacrifices to see this book written in a short time. Chris Towner typed the entire book and its hundreds of afterthoughts at record-breaking speed to meet a near-impossible deadline. She used a computer, although she had never touched one before—and all in her spare time or holiday. She sorted out the never-ending jumble of pages, comments, and footnotes with amazing precision and thoroughness.

Ian Farquhar stepped in at short notice to relieve me of a huge project while Ian Brown and others took over various other responsibilities. Dr Edwin Chilvers kindly interrupted his own busy writing schedule to loan his computer. He also provided helpful comments and insights.

I am indebted to Gerald Coates for his practical support, care, encouragement, and shaping of priorities. His emphasis on relationships, openness, honesty, integrity, and community involvement has influenced my life and this book, which led to the setting up of AIDS Care Education and Training (ACET) as a channel of practical help for those in need. Dr Caroline

Collier, AIDS officer of the Christian Medical Fellowship, was of great help in directing me towards good sources of information and in debating difficult ethical issues. Caroline Akehurst of the AIDS unit at the Bureau of Hygiene and Tropical Diseases does a magnificent job with limited resources, producing various information services and bulletins on AIDS.

Dr George Rutherford, director of the AIDS unit in San Francisco, and his secretary Ann Schlegel, were of immense help during my visit there.

I am indebted to Help the Hospices for kindly sponsoring the visit, and to Professor Eric Wilkes for his insistence that I should go and see the situation for myself and for helping to sort out funding at short notice.

Dr Veronica Moss of Mildmay Mission Hospital helped provide useful information before I went. Bea Roman, director of development of the Shanti Project in San Francisco, contributed enormously to my understanding of the human toll of AIDS in the United States. The AIDS office of the Episcopal cathedral was also very helpful. Dr Elizabeth Ankers provided some first-hand insights into the African situation, as well as several useful anecdotes. Dr Naz Pambakian helped in all kinds of practical ways and contributed toward my understanding of various situations in London. Professor Michael Adler helped sort out some of the complexities of sero-prevalence rates. Dr Rob George has been a helpful friend and encourager. There are countless others I would like to thank but cannot name who have contributed stories and information—or just talked about what it is like to be dying of AIDS or to lose a good friend.

I owe a lot to St Christopher's Hospice and to all who have pioneered excellence in hospice care under Dame Cicely Saunders OBE. It was they who first fired my enthusiasm for the care of the dying. I spent four weeks there working on the wards as a nursing auxiliary when I was a medical student on one of their residential courses. It was a life-changing experience. Dr Hanratty, medical director of St Joseph's Hospice in Hackney, has been a great influence on me and showed me the practical aspects of good pain control. It was he, along with the nursing Sisters, who convinced me that care of the dying would not become overwhelmingly depressing but was a most amazing privilege. I learned it is deeply satisfying as well as worthwhile.

I am indebted to Jill Highet, Julia Franklin, Margaret Vincent, Joyce Bell, Dr Irene Higginson, and Dr Tobias for showing me what it is to be part of a truly multi-disciplinary team—without a leader but with a real sense of belonging and mutual commitment. I have appreciated their interest, encouragement, expertise, knowledge, and tolerance when I have sometimes seemed a little preoccupied.

Most of all a tribute is due to my wife, Sheila, as well as to our children, John, Caroline, Elizabeth and Paul. They have put up with a major disruption of family life while I have been doctoring, attending church commitments, or closeting myself away with pen, paper, and computer printouts. Sheila is always encouraging and supportive, even when it has meant taking risks and sacrificing time together. Without her not a page of this book would have been written and none of it would have been checked properly.

I am also especially grateful to Corinne Hendry and Sara Cole of ACET who helped enormously in checking and updating the material for this revised international edition.

A number of people have read parts of the manuscript at various stages and made innumerable comments and suggestions of which the majority have been incorporated into the book. However, the responsibility for the content is mine.

INTRODUCTION

Don't Tell People the Truth

Many people are scared of telling the truth about AIDS. They say it will cause panic.

My experience is that people respect you for being honest. No one believes you if you deliberately play down risks. You lose all credibility when you give the impression something is safe and someone dies after doing it. Common sense tells people that certain things must carry some risk.

After the Chernobyl disaster Soviet leaders tried to dispel panic by playing down the danger. It caused further panic. People felt they could not trust official news at all. The only thing that would have defused the situation was detailed, clear, accurate information such as daily radiation checks in all public areas verified by respected members of the community and clear information about radiation and signs of overdosage. The government soon realised this and started to produce clear, up-to-date information with geiger counters to measure radiation on all vegetables sold in the marketplace and regular tests of homes.

It is stupid to say that if you follow guidelines you cannot catch the virus causing AIDS from looking after someone with the disease. Accidents happen. Guidelines may be hard to follow in all situations and they may have to be modified in the future in the light of experience. People know there are risks in nursing a person with AIDS. There must be. Anyone knows that. What is needed is to convince people that when you say these risks are very small you can really be trusted, that you are not just kidding people to blackmail them into doing something you know might be dangerous. When people really trust that you are telling the truth, the whole truth, and nothing but the truth—then they see what the risks really are and feel secure in knowing what they are dealing with. Knowing the truth allows them to make intelligent decisions about what to do.

I'm going to tell the truth as best I can.

So that you can check things out for yourself, many references appear at the back of the book. These are in a shorthand that any librarian can understand. Sufficient information is given to turn to the exact pages of scientific publications. For reasons of space, authors' names and titles of papers have usually been omitted. Newspapers are from the UK unless otherwise stated. Day but not page is given.

Not everything is referenced. Sometimes a figure or comment has been jotted down and used later although I cannot remember the source. Sometimes the source has been a personal interview. Where I want to protect the person's identity the reference is 'personal communication'. Many reference materials can be ordered from your local library or the librarian can advise you further. Student friends, doctors, or nurses will have access to much larger libraries.

1

The Extent of the Nightmare

It was 1981. In a Los Angeles doctor's office the men sitting in white coats were worried: within a few weeks they had diagnosed their fourth case of a condition so incredibly rare they had hardly expected to see it in their collective professional lifetime. They were baffled by the series of strange pneumonias that got worse despite normal antibiotics. All of the patients were men. All were young. All of them had died.

Three and a half thousand miles to the east, at a hospital in New York, several doctors were faced with a similar problem: strange tumors and lethal pneumonias in young men. What was going on?

The cases were all reported to the infectious disease centre. Could this be some sort of epidemic? Were the pneumonias and cancers caused by the same thing? What did the men have in common? Every day new reports of deaths came flooding in.[1] It was becoming clear that most, if not all, of the deceased were men who had had sex with other men. The disease quickly became labeled 'the gay plague'.

Dozens of strange infections were seen—with all the classic signs of weakened natural defences. The disease was called AIDS—Acquired Immune Deficiency Syndrome. It took some time to discover that the culprit was a tiny virus, called the Human Immunodeficiency Virus or HIV. It is now known that someone can be infected with HIV for ten years or more before developing the illness called AIDS.

Just five years later, by November 1986, 15,345 people had already died, another twelve thousand were dying, and a further 120,000 were feeling unwell.[2]

People were realising that maybe another million people in the United States were also infected but were not yet ill.[3] At first the 'experts' predicted only one in ten of those infected would die, then two in ten, then three in ten, then nine out of ten.[4] Now some are saying everyone with the infection will die.[5]

Most estimates from the early 1980s were exceeded. By April 1990 in the United States there were over 126,000 cases reported. Most had already resulted in death and there were estimates of possibly 200,000 to 300,000 feeling unwell and maybe one million infected, representing over one in sixty of all men in the United States between the ages of twenty and fifty. In New York, AIDS is now the most common cause of death in women aged twenty-five to thirty-four,[6] and one in every sixty-one babies is carrying the virus. By 1992 some say there will be at least 145,000 people dying of AIDS in the United States, compared with only 26,000 in 1986.[7]

The number of people already doomed in the United States makes the Vietnam tragedy look like a minor skirmish. The soldiers' coffins, if placed end to end, would stretch for one thousand miles.[8] Yet all the time another similar but far more catastrophic disaster was silently destroying another continent, and no one had noticed.

The African experience

Some years after AIDS was first diagnosed in the United States, the first cases were recognised in Africa. Hindsight shows that for years thousands had been dying,[9] but their deaths were blamed on tuberculosis and other diseases.

In some parts of Central Africa, up to a fifth of all young women and their babies are now thought to be infected. Whole villages are being wiped out. A third of the truck drivers running the main north/south routes[10] and half the prostitutes in many towns are infected.[11] In some hospitals between eight and twenty-three pints of blood out of one hundred are infected with HIV. One relief agency has talked unofficially about pulling out of Central Africa. 'What's the point in drilling more wells when most of the people will be dead in a few years?'[12] The World Health Organisation says 5 million are infected.

Grandmothers are looking after their grandchildren because so many young men and women, the parents, have been wiped out by AIDS. Armies of troops in Central Africa are being depleted— not by rockets and machine guns, but by AIDS. African countries could become destabilised as their forces of young men become too ill to fight.[13] Breadwinners for families and providers of the countries' wealth are missing. The educated élite living in the main towns and cities have been worst hit. In the country, fields are uncultivated and cattle wander aimlessly.[14] Hospitals are crowded with patients lying in corridors and on floors. In clinics, many are emaciated and too weak to move. In Africa they call it the 'slim' disease. Some Africans believe if you sleep with only fat women you are safe. 'To be fat is to be healthy.'

Officials stand at the doors of some hospitals selecting the fit ones for treatment. Anyone who looks thin and weak is sent back into the bush—'Probably got AIDS; nothing we can do for him.' Many are sent away with perfectly treatable diseases such as tuberculosis.[15] You cannot tell the difference at the door. Years and years of careful preventive medicine is being undermined. How do you start educating about a disease which produces no illness for years when nurses are still battling against ingrained habits just to get mothers to give their children a healthy diet?

The children's wards are full of dying children. Many are babies under one or two years old. They are not dying of famine, but of AIDS. A terrible tragedy is that many caught the virus not while in their mothers' wombs, but from the use of unsterilised needles.[16] Imagine a nuclear disaster which wiped out all fifty-three million people in the United Kingdom. A television news report suggested that the toll in Africa could exceed seventy-five million people.[17] The problem is that by the time a country identifies 10,000 cases it can have 500,000 infected. We must educate now.[18]

I visited central Africa recently on an education project. Our team spoke to over twenty thousand people about basic health protection. Education can be very effective.[19]

AIDS is *not* a gay plague; there are thousands and thousands more women and children dying of AIDS throughout the world than there are gay men. It gained this reputation in the United States because gay men were first to be diagnosed. Right now HIV is spreading like wildfire through communities of drug addicts in the United States, to their husbands, wives, lovers, children, and out into the wider community. Sadly, too, many men, women and children have been infected from medical treatments—mainly from receiving blood or blood products prior to 1985. In other parts of the world there are eight to ten million people infected with HIV, and at least one million of them will have AIDS by 1994, and six million by 2000.[20]

The experience in the United Kingdom

The first reported case of AIDS in the United Kingdom was in 1981.[21] Today if you meet five gay men in a London bar, the chances are that one of them is infected, although he probably does not know it. He may also have felt ill recently but put it down to some odd viral disease. He was right. He is beginning to experience the first symptoms of AIDS. All five may still be having sex with men (and maybe wives or other women too). In two years the numbers infected at a London clinic went up from four out of one hundred to a staggering twenty-one out of a hundred.[22] When you know that one in five of your possible partners could infect you, you start rethinking your behaviour. It is this terrible statistic that began to change gay lifestyles, not the government campaign that started two years later. After all, if you knew that one in five of the people you went out with were positive, wouldn't it make you think again about 'safer sex' or sleeping with them at all?

By 1986 the numbers had risen from twenty-one to twenty-four out of one hundred. Another study suggests that the true figure is now nearer thirty-three out of one hundred[23]—slowing down but not yet stopped. How much higher can it go? Some groups of gay men in San Francisco now have infection rates higher than seventy out of one hundred.[24] The trouble is that once it gets this high people can become fatalistic, thinking they are probably already infected. They do not want to be tested so the few who are not infected yet may become so.[25] A recent survey showed that homosexuals in New York had reduced risky behaviour, but there was no increase in total abstinence.[26]

In Edinburgh, an estimated fifteen hundred people were infected in less than eighteen months through sharing dirty needles. Because a drug habit is expensive, many female drug injectors turn to prostitution to obtain drugs. As a result, half of the prostitutes in Edinburgh are now infected with HIV. In London, one in a hundred of *heterosexual* men and women attending sex disease clinics are carrying HIV.[27]

At the beginning of 1989 there were already more than nine thousand people ill in the United Kingdom as a result of the HIV infection. Many had no idea why they were feeling so unwell. One in ten had reached the stage of full-blown AIDS. The British government said that forty thousand or more were infected as early as March 1987. Others have since revised figures downwards.[28] By the end of 1989 there were at least thirty thousand people infected in the United Kingdom. Government estimates were that *twenty-five or more new people a day were being infected*.[29] Most new infection today is likely to be among those sharing dirty needles. Heterosexual spread is also growing.

If the interval between infection and death were only six weeks, the list of deaths each week would cover the back page of *The Times*. These were the statistics in the United Kingdom at the end of June 1990:

- 1,864 deaths from AIDS
- 3,433 reported cases of AIDS
- 12,000 feeling unwell
- 30,000 infected with HIV

It is now thought that at least 95 per cent of the thirty thousand infected with HIV will develop symptoms of AIDS. As has been shown, many have suggested that all who develop early symptoms eventually die of full-blown AIDS. Consider that only three thousand five hundred cases had occurred in San Francisco when I visited in 1987. There are possibly six times that number in and around London. The British government expects four thousand deaths from AIDS in the next three years (three times the current number). In 1987 a senior official at the Department of Health said he expected only 30 per cent of those infected with HIV to develop AIDS, while unofficially he thought everyone infected was going to die. Now in released statements, officials admit that most of those infected are likely to die.

In the United Kingdom life insurance premiums have tripled for young men and doubled for young women because of AIDS.[30] Some people will say, 'Yes, but I'm not gay and I'm not an addict, so I'm not at risk.' An American study showed that 70 per cent of gay men reported having sex with a woman in the previous three to four years.[31]

Women are becoming infected from men with and without using condoms. Condoms reduce the risk enormously but not completely. Heterosexual spread of AIDS is now happening in many western and central American countries, not just in Africa.

Although special reasons may be found why HIV has spread in Africa so widely, even outside Africa HIV behaves just like any other sexually-transmitted infection. And the behaviour of heterosexual men and women has been slow to change. During all the campaigning, sexually-transmitted diseases rose by 30 per cent in one London hospital among heterosexual men, and only one in ten were interested in using condoms.[32]

Doctors, nurses and dentists are becoming infected from patients they treat—usually following needlestick injuries—although the risk from such accidents is very low.[33] Children are becoming infected from being molested by their infected fathers.[34] Organ transplants have infected people.[35] More than twelve hundred people in the United Kingdom—two hundred and fifty of whom were children—were infected from medical treatments before proper precautions were taken.

The majority of these children have haemophilia, a bleeding disorder requiring regular blood transfusions. Until recently all of the blood was obtained from the United States. Although the British government had been warned that blood from the US could give people in the UK AIDS, they did not act immediately. By the end of March 1990, over thirty people had become infected with HIV from blood transfusions.[36] The United Kingdom became largely self-sufficient in blood products after a new laboratory costing £60 million (about 100 million dollars) was opened on April 29, 1987.[37]

In the United States, government and church estimates show that up to one third of all fifty-seven thousand Roman Catholic priests could be infected, and one high-ranking Anglican has said that he expects a similar proportion of United States Anglican clergy to be at risk also.

A US health official said, 'I and most of the public health directors I've talked to about this subject estimate that in our communities at least a third of Catholic priests under forty-five are homosexuals, and most are sexually active. They always engage in anonymous encounters, the highest risk sex of all, and when they want help they don't come to the clinics.'[38] Personal communication from a high-ranking church official in San Francisco gave the same figures. At least twelve priests in the United States have full-blown AIDS: some have been thrown out of the church; others have been hidden away.[39]

A recent survey of fifteen hundred United States Roman Catholic priests revealed that 20 per cent are homosexually inclined and 10 per cent are sexually active. However surveys often underestimate due to the dishonesty of participants.

The highest-ranking cleric to die of AIDS so far is a Methodist bishop in Texas. No one knows how he got infected. In the United Kingdom *The Times* has estimated that more than 100 Anglican clergy are already known to be positive.[40] Several priests have already died from AIDS.

An Anglican vicar quoted a doctor recently in saying that at least twenty clergy had full-blown AIDS. His own research suggests that 400 Anglican clergy belong to the Gay Christian Movement.[41]

Some parts of the church in the United States and the United Kingdom are experiencing phenomenal growth as part of what some have called restoration and renewal. Thousands of young people across the country are becoming Christians each year. Often there are spectacular conversions resulting in radical changes in lifestyle.[42] Heroin addicts throw away their needles. Marriages are rebuilt. Practising homosexuals cease their activity. The results are often permanent—but so is the previous infection. AIDS could destroy churches physically, emotionally, psychologically, and spiritually—unless they are prepared.

At a recent conference for church leaders, I met a man who had been a drug addict before his conversion four or five years ago. He is now leading a church. This is happening all over the country. Some of these people will develop AIDS. The conference had representatives from sixty or so churches of a wide variety of denominations. Three different church leaders came to me saying they had long-standing members of their congregations who were infected with HIV or who were dying of AIDS. None of the three individuals was gay and none was from London or Edinburgh. Two were former drug addicts from the Midlands and one was a child on the south coast.

So what do we do? How can we prevent the disease? How can we cure it? How can we cope with it? The rest of this book addresses these four questions. But is AIDS really so different from any other disease, or is it just the mass hysteria and panic associated with it?

What is so special about AIDS?

At a recent major medical conference there was an argument: Is there anything special about AIDS or not?

In one sense there is not. AIDS is just the latest in a long series of epidemics spread by sex. The number of people with sexually transmitted diseases attending clinics has risen threefold over the last fifteen years. There are now half a million new cases a year in the United Kingdom.[43] Sleeping around has always carried risks to health. Now it is becoming suicidal.

More than three hundred years ago a plague broke out in Europe and spread across the western world. Vast numbers died. Early symptoms were mild, the second stage made people very ill, and half of those who developed the third stage died, many with brain damage. It was a terrible disease, and it was spread by sex. It was named *syphilis*.

Syphilis only stopped being a major threat with the discovery of penicillin at the end of World War II. During the war, United States army recruits were warned that, after Hitler, syphilis was Public Enemy Number One.[44] Syphilis has not gone away; we are in the middle of a major heterosexual explosion of cases which often produce few or no symptoms and are untreated for a long period.

Gonorrhea also became a curable sexual disease with penicillin—until the recent advent of penicillin-resistant strains which are now spreading rapidly across the globe and becoming harder and harder to treat. There is an unprecedented epidemic of genital herpes. Highly infectious, appallingly painful blisters prevent sex. (Fourteen thousand cases are reported every year in the United Kingdom and the numbers are rising.[45]) There is no cure and it can cause problems throughout a person's life. There is also a big increase in cancer of the neck of the womb (cervix), some of which is associated with a virus infection and is due to sleeping with multiple partners.

There is also the heart-rending problem of infertility. Have you ever wondered about the huge test-tube baby programme? As a medical student I remember attending the ward rounds of an obstetrics professor. He used to joke about a colleague who filled the ward with his infertile patients. He could tell which patients were his colleague's and not his own—his colleague's patients were the good-looking ones! The major part of his colleague's workload was people with badly damaged and scarred fallopian tubes – the thin delicate tubes which guide the egg from the ovary to the womb. The cause was an infection called pelvic inflammatory disease (PID), which can be caused by a tiny organism called *chlamydia*.[46] There is no treatment that can undo the damage of pelvic inflammatory disease. One in ten women develop it after being infected with chlamydia, gonorrhea, or some other infections. It causes aches and pains that are chronically disabling, and it gradually causes the reproductive organs to stick together.

Then came a new disease—AIDS—that many people think has been around in Africa, the US and Europe for decades before recognition in the late 1980s.[47] Wherever it started, it spread slowly at first, undetected, and then explosively among men, women, and young children. It was only detected as it hit the medical technology of the United States, was misdiagnosed as an American gay curiosity, and only traced to its probable roots some two or three years later.[48]

The difference between HIV-related diseases and other sexual epidemics is that HIV can infect you for years before you know it, and by the time you do it has spread to infect possibly hundreds of others. The other difference is that once you develop full-blown AIDS—which can take many years—you face certain death. There is no cure and no vaccine, nor is either anywhere in sight. There are many misleading reports but no good results.

A rapidly-spreading, silent killer which is difficult to detect, infectious, and lethal causes panic. Radiation disasters are similar: you cannot hear, see, feel, or touch the enemy, nor feel the damage it is doing until too late—sometimes not for years. No wonder the Chernobyl disaster caused such terrible pandemonium: false rumours, false scares, false cures, false hopes abounded. AIDS is the same today.

If a man had sex with his secretary and three weeks later was dead, and that was repeated across the country, the impact would be dramatic. You would not need any health campaign because the coffins would be the campaign. But with HIV and AIDS the enormous time lag produces a credibility problem: the only people who really understand what is likely to hit us are the mathematicians. An invisible terror can be ignored.

If we have to wait ten years to see exactly what is happening, we will be too late. We need to learn now from what is going on in San Francisco.

San Francisco: the shape of things to come?

By mid-1987 in San Francisco, nearly three thousand five hundred people had been diagnosed as having AIDS. Just over 1,000 were still alive, with probably 10,000 others in a city of 800,000 already feeling unwell, and maybe 100,000 infected.[49]

Most gay men I talked with had buried between ten and twenty of their friends. A grandmother broke down and wept as she told me that her five-year-old grandson was dying. He had always been a somewhat sickly child, full of coughs and colds. One day he developed a rare chest infection and the doctors did an HIV antibody test: it was positive. They tested his mother and found that she was positive too. She was perfectly well but had led a somewhat risky life before she got married. She was devastated. Even now she cannot accept the doctor's diagnosis. The son of the woman I was talking to was fortunately still negative. She told me of another family she knew where Mum and Dad had both died, as had five of their children, one by one, until only the nine-year-old was left. 'She's doing fine, settled in her new school, with foster parents. She has got AIDS, of course, and she knows it, but she's a plucky little girl.' I found I was crying too.

During my stay in San Francisco I began to realise the overwhelming tragedy of the disease. I began to see why nurses and volunteers reach the point where they cannot go on. Many of them are personally involved: maybe they have recently nursed a friend with AIDS, or maybe they think they are positive themselves.

The same has happened in the United Kingdom. On one ward close to a third of the male nurses are infected because of personal lifestyles.[50] Others may have personal experience of the disease. It is understandable: cancer hospices have always drawn staff and volunteers from those who have been bereaved. However, hospices have known the dangers of giving in to pressures to accept help too soon. The recently bereaved soon find themselves reliving their own tragedy with every patient they see. Often the resulting grief and turmoil become overwhelming. They leave the ward in tears, have unpleasant dreams, are unable to sleep, or become convinced that they too are developing the disease. A complete break from this kind of work is usually essential to prevent serious depression. This can be hard if supporting friendships, identity, and meaning in life are also tied up with the hospice.

I saw the same thing happening in San Francisco on a grand

scale: whole communities becoming overloaded with grief, except that this is grief of a different kind.[51] With AIDS there is the second sinister dimension: if you become part of an AIDS ward team or volunteer programme because of nursing a lover with AIDS, there is the terrible possibility that you yourself are also infected with HIV. Not only do you then relive awful memories of the one you cared for as he died with each patient, but there is the hideous reality at the forefront of your mind that tomorrow it may be your turn. Every time you take a shower you find yourself checking all over for telltale signs of Kaposi's sarcoma—a form of skin cancer associated with AIDS. Every cough, cold, or fever becomes a clanging bell of disaster. Every episode of diarrhoea or feeling tired becomes a living nightmare. Every act of forgetfulness becomes a warning of dementia.

Sheer fright can produce the entire symptoms of early infection. A doctor in New York was convinced he had AIDS after a minor incident. He worried, became depressed and tired, stopped eating, and lost weight. He had diarrhoea, produced a temperature, and finally developed rashes typical of early infection. Every test was negative—even the HIV antibody test. He then became convinced that he was in the one or two out of one hundred who never produce a positive test. This man has been followed up. He did not have AIDS or any other early signs, and his immune system is completely normal.[52]

A nurse, doctor or volunteer can find he is daily helping people dying of AIDS, supporting a colleague who is now becoming ill but wants to continue working (despite early signs of deteriorating brain function, encephalopathy), and then to cap it all, going home to nurse a dying lover of several years' standing. AIDS, AIDS, AIDS. No wonder so many are under a lot of stress. When you have already been to ten funerals of friends in the last year, you can reach the point of not coping any longer.

Then there is the terrible dilemma: what do you do when your colleague is becoming forgetful, clumsy and slowing up mentally? He is probably only too aware of what is happening and why. In one out of ten people this can be the first sign of

AIDS.[53] Are you going to put him on permanent sick leave? Sick pay starts to run out after six months and stops after a year.[54] The person needs income and a stabilising routine. If you were to ask me what the first sign of encephalopathy is I would say it could be something like a pilot attempting to land with no undercarriage in place. I understand that British Airways is so worried about subtle loss of mental performance in airline pilots that it now routinely screens new pilots for HIV.[55] They have reason to be worried: nine of its male stewards are already dead and thirty-one more have full-blown AIDS.[56] A British newspaper published the nine death certificates because nobody believed the newspaper story.[57] DanAir includes HIV antibody tests as a routine part of the regular 'medicals' on cabin crew.[58]

A nursing organisation in the United States of America is thinking of introducing special intelligence tests for staff. When performance drops below a certain level they will be suspended from duty and will probably be fired.[59] With patient workload doubling every year they cannot afford to carry an increasing number of mentally deteriorating staff on their payroll.

At the moment the gay community in San Francisco provides most of the volunteers. But the gay community will soon be overwhelmed, with many volunteers dead and vast numbers unwell.[60] Fewer and fewer well people will be left to look after more and more who are dying. The same will be true of New York and London unless many more volunteers are recruited from outside the gay community. London hospital staff are already showing signs of severe stress due to heavy workloads and the intense nature of the disease.[61] Another problem is that it is very unusual to find supportive networks of friends around infected drug addicts.

One of the AIDS experts I met was shaking like a leaf. In the course of the one-hour interview it became clear that he was yet another person experiencing multiple losses: his lover had died at home recently, people in the office were ill or had died, and he had been to more than twelve funerals. He had no problems thinking, but his nerves were damaged by HIV, hence the uncontrollable shake.

If San Francisco faces a crisis, New York faces a catastrophe since it has many more residents, many drug users and other groups without the emotionally supportive networks seen on the West Coast. The state of New York will have to play a much larger role in caring for those ill. Already by 1989, over two thousand hospital beds were full on any given day because of HIV,[62] with a projected increase to 4,000 per day in 1994.

Why San Francisco became a gay centre

In San Francisco I was welcomed by a senior churchman who was dying of AIDS. He explained to me how Europeans sailed west two hundred years ago to get away from persecution in Europe and landed on the East Coast. Those who could not settle there drifted into the great plains. Those uncomfortable there drifted further west to the Rockies. Beyond the Rockies lay eight hundred miles of arid desert and beyond that lay the dream: San Francisco. A tiny collection of Spanish huts in the early nineteenth century, it was overtaken by the Gold Rush of the 1840s and then by the discovery of silver lode in the desert. A vast town sprang up where people risked and lost, loved and died.

A free-wheeling fantasy world was shattered by the vast earthquake of 1904 which destroyed four square miles and killed thousands of people. The new San Francisco was built over the ashes of the terrible fire that followed. The rebuilt city was populated by those 'going West', by Chinese from the East, and by immigrants from the South.

Part of the American dream has always been to opt out and escape by 'going West'. San Francisco was the centre for the beatniks of the 1950s and then the hippie movement of the 1960s. 'Make love not war' was the motto for prolonged anti-Vietnam demonstrations and drug-using 'free love' communes. The bubble burst in the 1970s with violence related to drug offenders. But then came a new migration West of people who felt they were unaccepted further East: homosexual men and women.

San Francisco has always had a reputation for carefree living, tolerance, and sexual freedom—especially after the hippies came, cut their hair, and settled down. Once a gay community was established, it grew rapidly. The gay districts used to be some of the poorest areas of downtown San Francisco, now they are becoming more fashionable. Gay consciousness became an important political force so that by the early 1980s it commanded 25 per cent of the vote at elections for mayors and other local government officers.[65] Then the latest bubble was burst by a tiny virus.

The great cover-up

Why are so few people being honest about the extent of the problem and the risks? The first area of cover-up is in government because of intolerance and tightly controlled health budgets. In San Francisco people in the gay community talk of 'passive genocide' that they feel was practised by former President Reagan's administration for six or seven years. The problem of AIDS was barely acknowledged. Some have said that Reagan failed to implement in full the recommendations of his comimssion on the HIV epidemic, in particular on the issue of discrimination.[66] Reagan was quoted as talking about infected children as 'the innocent sufferers', so by implication the rest are guilty. American society has always been rather intolerant of 'non-survivors' of the system. Those who are unemployed, chronically sick, or cannot afford health insurance are often in a desperate plight. The intolerance is especially magnified for problems considered to be directly related to a person's own decisions. Poverty is often considered to be the result of laziness. Diseases spread by sexual practices or drug abuse are condemned. There is a strong undercurrent of anti-homosexual feeling. Several conservative religious groups that helped elect Reagan are controlled by immensely powerful people with colossal grassroots support. Some of them are known for right-wing statements, on apartheid for example, but more recently for declaring that AIDS is the wrath of God on homosexuals. Elsewhere in this book, these comments are examined and found to be unreasonable and absurd, particularly in view of what is now known of the disease in Africa. In some parts of the United States the feeling has been that homosexuals and drug addicts are being wiped out (at last). The momentum to educate, plan, or treat them has been negligible.

This partly explains why the United States, faced in 1988 with an unavoidable national disaster—barring a new miracle cure—has only recently leafleted every home[67] or considered advertising condoms on TV. The point has only come now because the disease threatens other groups of people. The whole nation is now felt to be at risk.

Apart from the national lack of interest in what happens to gays or drug addicts, there has been a pressing economic reason for a great cover-up. In the early days when strange pneumonias and skin diseases were first noticed, these things plus several other strange infections were called AIDS. Unless you had one of these things you did not have AIDS. Even when the virus was discovered and people could be tested for antibodies, those who were positive and unwell could not be classified as having AIDS. Even if they were clearly dying as a result of the infection, they could not be labelled 'AIDS patients' if they did not have a second infection or tumor that counted.[68]

Clearly the definition has become meaningless. You can be either infected and feeling well, or infected and feeling ill. The sicker you get, the more likely it is you will die soon. However, the original, inadequate definition remains and will continue to remain, with occasional minor extensions. Why? Because of money and politics.

The federal government will only allow certain benefits to be given, including free supplies ($6,500 per person) of Zidovudine (AZT) to those who 'officially' have AIDS. AZT is the major drug used to slow down HIV in the body. The federal government may end this subsidy soon, meaning people with AIDS will have to stop treatment or face bankruptcy.[69] All the statistics collected are for AIDS. Yet for every person who fits the AIDS definition, another ten are feeling ill, so the problem is at least ten times worse than statistics show.[70]

The second area of cover-up is among those whose lives have

been devastated by AIDS. People who should be able to kick up a fuss about it are those whose friends and lovers are desperately ill without being labelled as having AIDS. They will not complain because they cannot. When I mentioned the problem to a group of volunteers in San Francisco there was a strong reaction. The people there are so overloaded with grief and stress they can hardly conceive how they will cope next year with double the numbers of people with AIDS and four times the year after and eight times the year after that. They are unable to cope with the thought that HIV may already be affecting the health of ten times as many as the people they know of. 'Please don't say that,' said one person. 'We can hardly bear what we are seeing now. If we even stop to think about ARC (early AIDS), we will just cave in.'

So here are people who could challenge the government's estimates but are inadequate for the task because they are so overwhelmed emotionally that they too are helping to play down the situation.

Another area where those closest to the problem are numbed into silence is in the problem of encephalopathy, or deterioration of the brain. In San Francisco and elsewhere, doctors are becoming better at treating strange chest infections and other illnesses. The length of life of someone newly diagnosed with full-blown AIDS is longer than it was. But now the more hideous problem of encephalopathy is emerging. When examined after death, brains of people with AIDS all show significant damage due to destruction of brain cells by the virus.[71] Sometimes this has been obvious during life, sometimes not. The brain damage can impair thinking, alter personality, change behaviour, rob people of dignity, and even affect movement. With careful testing it now seems that some evidence of mental deterioration can probably be found in most people who are about to die as a result of AIDS.[72] It is a terrible nightmare when you see it develop in your best friend, your colleagues, and in yourself.

Remember that many people working in these projects at the moment know that their own lifestyle means they are quite likely to be infected already. Being faced with possible progressive brain damage is so horrific that many people are unable to accept it. A state of denial is common in people with cancer and here we are seeing denial in AIDS health care workers and decision makers.

A third area of denial or cover up is in discussions of the numbers of people likely to go on to develop full-blown AIDS. Statements that only ten out of one hundred would do so soon looked absurd, given the rate at which the numbers were increasing and the nature of the virus. Indeed the estimate was revised a year or so later to twenty out of one hundred. These figures persisted for years, being trotted out again and again.

One of the problems has been continued circulation of out-of-date leaflets that contain no date of publication. The proportion of those infected who were developing AIDS was clearly still increasing rapidly so why didn't people say so? Soon the figures were revised again, and so on. The increases became obvious, inevitable, predictable—so why the strangely optimistic statements?

A senior official of the United Kingdom Department of Health told me unofficially that if he were honest he thought the final numbers dying—say after fifteen years—would be nearer 100 per cent. The official version at the same time was a mere thirty-five or so out of one hundred, with the possibility of more. I think part of the reason was a desire to give as much hope as possible to those who were infected. Some of the people I met who quoted research papers so confidently were themselves infected. Seizing on these low estimates is a further kind of denial: a way of coping with personal fears.

The same thing results in wild claims being made for new drugs. 'Dementia won't be a problem now that we have AZT,' a senior AIDS counsellor told me two years ago. I wish that was what we were seeing at home and on the wards.

A fourth area of cover-up has been over the risks of infection by non-sexual, non-injecting contact. For example, statements have been widely circulated that HIV is very fragile and cannot survive except at body temperature for more than a few minutes.[73] It has also been said that it cannot withstand drying. These statements were made in good faith but were obviously wrong. Ask any haemophiliac who became infected from blood extracts. These extracts are obtained by freeze drying. The powder is then stored in a warehouse, transported to a hospital, and several weeks or months later it is reconstructed with sterile water before injection. The organisms causing gonorrhea or syphilis would be destroyed instantly by such harsh treatment. But people can be infected with HIV this way.

Researchers took samples of HIV and placed them on a number of dishes to dry. After a day, the first sample was tested to see if it was infectious, and it was. The second day's sample was also infectious—and so on, right up to the end of a week. Some of the virus survived in dry dust for up to seven days. Then they repeated the experiment using the virus in water. They took samples each day and found that even after two whole weeks in water a few virus particles remained capable of causing infection. The public had been told pasteurisation (fifty-six degrees Centigrade for twenty minutes) killed the virus, but this same research showed that heating to fifty-six degrees Centigrade must be continued for at least three hours to destroy all virus particles.[74]

This research has been criticised. The amount of virus used was enormous. If the smaller amounts found in blood had been used, the results would probably have been different. The study is being repeated. In spite of this criticism it is still quite extraordinary that such a potentially important paper received so little attention, as it has vast implications for public health.

Although the study was included in Great Britain's Department of Health (DH) circular on preventing cross-infection,[75] it has not been widely reported. I think the reason is that medical personnel are scared that if everyone knew about it they would be even more reluctant to look after those with AIDS. A member of the DH said the report had 'set the cat among the pigeons'. Sixty thousand copies were distributed to all the health districts in the United Kingdom, yet hardly anyone has seen it. The DH found that all thirty copies sent to one district were put straight into a filing cabinet and forgotten.[76]

Likewise, other reports that break unspoken rules are not being given wide coverage. Doctors and nurses who have become infected are being kept out of the media's eye, as are a steady trickle of others who are being infected through unusual routes. At least six are already known to have become infected through skin contact with secretions or blood. The skin is full of special white cells, Langerhans macrophages and T-helper lymphocytes, which are particularly susceptible to infection by the virus if the skin is cracked or broken; intact skin is an excellent barrier to HIV. So the virus does not have to enter blood, but only the deeper skin layers.[77]

However, to put it in context as you will see in other sections of this book, the risk even to medical personnel of becoming infected other than through sex or sharing dirty needles is incredibly small. It is just being pointed out that what has been said in public is often not the whole truth.

The fifth area of cover-up is the failure to acknowledge prominently two possible errors in all of the figures reported for full-blown AIDS.[78] We considered earlier the omission of up to ten times the numbers reported of those sick but not having full-blown AIDS. However, another problem is failure by doctors to report cases. Reporting is totally voluntary in the United Kingdom and the United States. Some diseases like smallpox must be reported by law so they can be investigated and contacts can be traced. But voluntary reporting is always, by its nature, incomplete. Reactions to drugs are supposed to be reported on a voluntary basis and yet I know—from being a busy junior doctor—that when you have twenty people waiting to be admitted to the ward to be prepared for operations the following day, reports that are not essential to patient safety and care today tend to get put off until tomorrow. By the following week the details have been mislaid or seem less important—'After all, what is one report among so many? It won't make any great difference.' A few weeks later the report still has not been sent in. 'Where shall I send it? What is the address?' Sometimes doctors may assume that someone else has already done it anyway.

The second possible source of underestimating the numbers of AIDS cases is incorrect diagnosis. As the spectrum of the disease widens, more and more doctors will be asking themselves if AIDS was not in fact the explanation for that curious death some time ago. An example is pneumonia. Despite antibiotics, and before AIDS, people still occasionally died of pneumonia. As people get older, it becomes a more common cause of death. In the elderly it is very common indeed. Most people with AIDS are young so chest infections are more conspicuous, but there is the possibility that some older people may be dying of unrecognised AIDS-related pneumonias.[79]

A second example is death from an accident caused by unrecognised early brain damage. Even where the correct diagnosis is made, AIDS is often not recorded on the death certificate in order to save relatives distress. Pneumonia is often put down as the cause. This is yet another way that cases may not land in the statistics even when diagnosed. A recent health department survey of young male deaths in the United Kingdom found a large unexplained increase. Examination of records suggests that many of these deaths were due to AIDS although not recognised at the time.[80] A sixth area of cover-up is the dishonesty of some who have become infected about how they came to be so. A man may say he slept with a prostitute once in 1983 but has otherwise been faithful to his wife. Several weeks later he admits he is a practising homosexual. Many of the 15 per cent listed with 'no known risk factors' fall into this area. An extreme example is in the United States armed forces where up to three-quarters can give no explanation or only a heterosexual one.[81] The general unease about being honest makes it extremely difficult to monitor different methods of spreading.

I am not suggesting that these areas of cover-up are all the result of deliberate conspiracy; some aspects may be, others are part of a poor system of communication, and still others are non-deliberate distortions of a complex, confusing, and rapidly-changing picture. However, they all add up to a situation where what the average doctor, nurse, or member of the public understands is often only a part of the whole problem.

The African cover-up

The distortion of the real problem in the United States or United Kingdom is negligible in comparison to the almost complete silence of some African governments. Confronted with a tragedy affecting their whole continent—and for once not related to war or famine—in an international atmosphere which they see as racist, many have been extremely unwilling to be honest. They are afraid of anti-black backlash if it is said that the problem started there. They are also afraid of economic ruin due to decisions of multinational companies to pull out, and the collapse of their tourist industries. Many of these countries desperately need foreign currency to prevent total bankruptcy. In addition it has often been difficult for doctors to be sure of the diagnosis. Testing is expensive, kits are hard to obtain, and sometimes hard to use. Indirect methods have to be used such as a negative skin reaction to the standard tuberculosis (TB) test.[82] Most AIDS-related deaths seem to be happening out in the bush, unnoticed and unregistered. The wards and clinics see mainly early cases.

So we have a bizarre situation where doctors in these countries are reeling under an impossible workload, and where even government members or relations of the country's leaders are dying,[83] but the problem is denied, or impossible to assess. Possibly twenty cases are admitted, or one hundred, or one thousand, or ten thousand. The statements are usually meaningless. Scientists studying the epidemic in Central Africa are there under tolerance. Intensive research is going on all over Africa to understand the disease, but the results are censored. A scientist will often have to sign an agreement not to disclose publicly what he sees happening. Information is leaking out all the time, but if it is traced back to a particular person or team the workers may be thrown out of the country or into prison. Fortunately, the situation is changing. It has to. The cover-up has had one appalling consequence which prevents an educational campaign. How can a country embark on mass prevention for a disease it says it does not really have? Once again we see denial for emotional reasons too, not just economic ones.

How can you accept from a mathematician that maybe a third of your entire nation could die?[84]

South Africa has its own reasons to cover up. It has an enormous problem, especially in the black townships where huge numbers of migrant workers come from countries further north in which AIDS is taking a terrible toll.

In places like Soweto, the town providing labour for the deep mines in Johannesburg, there are sometimes up to fifty thousand men living without their wives (officially). Their wives and children are all meant to stay in homelands like the Transkei. They don't, of course, and drift out in search of their husbands to build illegal residences made from corrugated iron, wood, and plastic. Every now and then these 'shanty towns' are bulldozed to the ground and the women trucked back, sometimes more than one thousand miles away.

Fifty thousand men on their own with a few prostitutes spells trouble—yet this situation is common in South Africa. The government has no political will to change anything. For them, a major disease that selectively hits black Africans and offsets the birthrate may be convenient. I doubt if we will see any major effective preventative campaign. However, South Africa is admitting an increasing problem in its white population. Since black prostitutes commonly serve white men—frowned on but it happens—they may be stirred into action this way.[85]

Eastern Europe is now admitting a huge problem. Official statistics from every country in the world are listed in Appendix D.

The church cover-up

Although Britain's Lesbian and Gay Christian movement says there could be as many as six thousand gay clergy in the United Kingdom, and although the number of clergy who are developing AIDS is steadily climbing,[86] the problem is not officially acknowledged.

To the non-churchgoing public it seems that at a time of inner crisis, the church reacts by closing ranks. No wonder clear definitive statements on family life and sexual behaviour have not been forthcoming, at least not until the appointment of the new Archbishop of Canterbury in July 1990.

In the United States the situation is further confused by many clergy's fear of discovery. This is not just a priest's fear of being recognised by a visitor or by the chaplain on an AIDS ward, but the fear that parishioners may suspect a hidden life-style.

At a recent Anglican conference in Washington, the church position on various issues relating to homosexuality was debated. A senior clergyman, who was a practising homosexual himself, told me how angry he had been to see priests whom he recognised from gay bars and other haunts voting in favour of harsh anti-homesexual statements.

Life after AIDS

Cover-up or no cover-up, honesty, secrecy, or confusion, one thing is clear: nothing will ever be quite the same again. AIDS will fundamentally alter fashions, behaviour, culture—in fact every fibre of our society. In New York, fat is back in fashion: 'Who wants to look thin—perhaps he has AIDS.' Who would have thought that in 1987 James Bond would be portrayed as having a stable relationship? Sex three times with the same woman, not once each with three women! The Hollywood dinosaur of the movie industry is thrashing its tail and the ground is shaking. Television producers are stepping over each other in their zeal to include AIDS in soap operas, plays, and comedies.[88]

Magazines like *Cosmopolitan* say that smart girls carry condoms. They hope that smart girls will not feel like loose girls when they produce the packet. They hope too for a new courage and honesty so that people will always tell of their unfaithfulness and promiscuity or drug addiction. They hope for new security in relationships so that when a girl or boy suggests using a condom, the other will not treat it as a terrible insult or lack of trust.

Whether such hopes will remain hopes or get built into a

strange harsh reality of rubber-separated sex is unclear. But one thing is certain: out of the ashes of the crematorium will rise a new sub-culture which will affect a whole generation: a culture of stable relationships and marriages. A culture where the macho man is the man who can fulfil his woman in every way for a lifetime.

The reality is that even an AIDS cure in 1995 or a remarkable vaccine in 1997 will not erase the traumas of a generation. The message is burning home: sleeping around has always been unhealthy. Now it is suicidal. Taking AIDS out still leaves the other epidemics untouched. The mid-twenty-first century will look at the 1980s, 1990s, and the early years of the next century as the 'era of AIDS'. The reasons for its spread, its origins, the apathy of governments, and the mistakes of scientists will be debated by historians for generations.

AIDS will dominate the rest of our adult lives—especially the lives of doctors and nurses. The question is this: will you be able to hold your head high? Will you be proud of the way you responded when you look back on it all?

Apart from a radical change of lifestyle in our society—which will not help those already infected anyway—our only hope remains in understanding this strange virus so we can fight it. But what exactly *is* a virus?

2

What's so Special about a Virus?

All viruses are dead. There is nothing alive in a virus at all. A virus is no more living than a computer game you can buy in the High Street. Bacteria are different: bacteria breathe oxygen or carbon dioxide, need warmth to grow, and they grow larger and divide into two. In fact bacteria behave like cells in your own body.

Some bacteria make poisons such as the tetanus toxin which causes rapid death. Others live quite happily on every corner of your body. An example is in your gut where bacteria help you to digest food. If you take antibiotics, some of these bacteria die and the result can be diarrhoea. So while some bacteria keep us healthy, others bring disease because of the poisons they make when growing.

You can see bacteria under the microscope. I have taken a swab from a man's penis or a woman's vagina and touched a microscope slide with it. You can see the red gonorrhoea bacteria easily and make an instant diagnosis. In most cases a single large dose of penicillin will kill all the bacteria. Penicillin works by weakening the cell wall that holds the little organism together. The bacteria swell, burst, and die. A swab containing syphilis organisms is even more interesting: these creatures swim like little eels, thrashing about on the wet glass slide. Instant diagnosis. Immediate high dose penicillin. Immediate cure in most cases.

But AIDS is caused by a virus (HIV).[1] Thousands of bacteria can fit inside a cell in your body, but virus particles are so minute that hundreds of thousands of them could fit inside a single bacterium. They are totally invisible under a normal light microscope. Viruses cannot grow and cannot divide. They don't breathe, don't need food, don't live, and never die. All our technology has failed to produce a single drug that attacks and destroys a virus directly.

The kiss of death

The only weapons we have against viruses are natural ones: antibodies which can also destroy bacteria. These are Y-shaped. The mouth of the antibody is shaped exactly to fit over part of a germ. Thousands of them lock onto a germ so that the tails bristle like a hedgehog. Sometimes that is enough to burst bacteria or to stop viruses from being able to touch a cell. Special white cells in the body stick on to these bristles and eat up the germ. These white cells are those that you find in pus, cleaning up an infected wound. The trouble with antibodies is that the body takes three days to produce the right antibody for the right virus. During this critical three-day period, the body is totally unprotected. Yet only an hour or two after viruses enter the bloodstream they have completely disappeared. You can hunt through the entire body, cell by cell, with the best electron-firing microscope and find nothing.

Why? Because every virus particle has disintegrated. Each one has burst like a soap bubble when it touches the ground.

The virus bag has disintegrated and vanished. What about the contents? They too have disappeared without trace, but the cell it touched has received the kiss of death.[2]

Diseases

Viruses	Bacteria
Colds	Boils
Flu	Pneumonias (most types)
Measles	Tuberculosis
Chickenpox/Shingles	Diphtheria
Polio	Tetanus
Herpes/cold sores	Cystitis
Smallpox	Food poisoning
Glandular fever	Gonorrhoea
Rabies	Syphilis
Hepatitis	
AIDS	

A sentence that kills

A virus is a bag containing a short piece of coiled up 'string'. The string is formed entirely of four different chemicals arranged in an order. When stretched out, it reads like a language:

ABBDA AABDACCC ABDA CCDAAAB AA CCDAA

This language is what we call a genetic code. It is the language used by the nucleus (brain) of every cell in your body. A cell of your body under the microscope looks a little like an egg. It has a central round core called a nucleus and a more transparent-looking outer area. The nucleus is black and is packed full of your chromosomes. You have forty-six chromosomes which determined everything from the moment you were conceived, including the length of your arms, whether you have black or brown hair, whether you will be bald by the time you are thirty, your height, gender, basic build, the shape of your nose. Everything.

Each of these chromosomes is tightly coiled up like a spring. If we stretched out the message and then typed out the sequence, and put all the messages from all the chromosomes in one cell from your body into a book, that book would be the size of *Encyclopaedia Britannica*.

These instructions programme not only your outside appearance, but also every type of cell in your body. Have you ever thought how a skin cell learned it was a skin cell and not a nail- or hair-producing cell? How does a cell know it should produce bone and not hormones? If I cut my hand, how does a skin cell know to divide and go on dividing until the gap is covered and then stop? The answer lies in that vast book of instructions. The amazing thing is that *every* cell nucleus in your body carries a carbon copy of your entire genetic code.

Sinister experiments

If I take the nucleus (core) out of a single skin cell of a frog, and take the nucleus out of an unfertilised frog's egg, and put into that transparent egg a black dot which is the nucleus of that skin cell, a remarkable thing happens which you can watch under the microscope. (The procedure is easy in frogs because their egg nuclei are so big.) As you watch you will see that egg cell divide into four, then eight, then sixteen and thirty-two and so on. At this early stage any one of these cells, if separated, could go on to produce a twin frog. If the cells are left in a ball, each senses the presence of its neighbours, reads its book of instructions, and starts to develop different behaviour. One cell goes on to produce the brain, another the spinal cord, and so on. The result is a clone of the frog we took the skin from.

We will very soon be able to do the same with human eggs. Scientists are very near being able to take a nucleus from a cell in my body, put it into an egg, and produce a clone or an identical twin of me. The only difference is that the twin will be years younger. The egg would develop to a full baby by being placed in the womb of a surrogate mother.

Deadly secrets

Some scientists hate talking about this kind of work. I found myself one evening eating with the research fellows of a particular college in England. After some wine, my neighbour at the table confessed that he was nearing his lifetime ambition: the ultimate in spare-part surgery.

He was able now, he claimed, to take a nucleus from his own body, put it into a human egg, place the egg in the womb of a monkey, and grow it to a foetus. 'Unfortunately' these foetuses were dying sooner than he would like. If only he could grow that foetus for a few weeks more he could 'cull' it, kill the monkey, kill the foetus and use—say—the young healthy kidneys of his murdered twin to replace his own. He was not publishing his work in this area because he was sure his laboratory would be closed down. His laboratory is extremely well known.[3]

I am telling you this for two reasons: first, to indicate how complex your genetic code is in every cell of your body, and second, to emphasise that as a race we are on the brink of terrible disaster—whether nuclear, biological as in AIDS, or through genetic tampering with life itself.

Life-changing technology

We have already succeeded in altering the genetic code of a bacterium so it contains a small piece of code taken from a human being: this piece of code tells the bacterium not to produce poison but to produce human insulin—previously diabetics were dependent on insulin obtained by crushing the pancreas of a pig or cow. This new strain of bacteria grows and divides forever, with each new organism containing a perfect set of instructions for making human insulin.

Scientists in the United States have just won the legal right to patent any new species they create by taking genetic code from one animal or plant and putting it into another. We have the technology now for creating cows which produce not cows' milk, but a perfect human-style baby milk. How about a tree that produces apples that taste like oranges, or a horse with the head and mischievousness of a monkey?[4]

Various laboratories around the world are locked into a race to 'decode' the entire genetic material of a human. This enables us to say that:

ABCADDA = Insulin;
BCADDDD = Length of nose;
BCCABBA = Amount of pigment in hair.[5]

The correct bit for any part of a human can then be cut out and transferred, or be reprogrammed and put back into the cell.

So then, it is also possible to map out every single instruction a virus contains and understand precisely what it does in the cell it affects. Why can't all this remarkable technology produce a cure for AIDS? Consider what happens when the virus bubble touches its target cell.

How the virus kills a white cell

The surface of HIV is specially shaped so that it only fits onto a very small range of cells in the body. The flu virus latches onto cells in the nose, while HIV mainly latches onto one particular type of white cell (T4), some brain cells, and one or two others.[6]

When HIV touches the cell and the bubble bursts, the genetic code is injected suddenly into the cell. Within minutes the code is being read by the cell and the message is being carried into the cell brain, or nucleus. The message is then added permanently to that cell's 'book of life'. The process took only a few minutes and is complete. The cell looks normal in every way but is now doomed. It may continue to look normal for several years. During this time the white cell continues to travel in the blood looking for invaders while blissfully unaware of the invader within. If the attacked cell divides, the two daughter cells also carry perfect copies of the hidden message.[7] It is likely that the infected cells in semen or vaginal fluids are the main source of HIV transmissions during sex.

Biological time-bomb

Each cell infected by HIV becomes a biological time-bomb travelling in the bloodstream. Millions of them waiting to explode.[8]

One day a particular germ enters the body that this particular cell is geared to deal with. There are thousands of different white cells, all designed to kill different kinds of organisms. It just so happens that out of all the thousands of different infections a person could have caught, this particular one fits the role of this particular cell. It springs into action, programmed by its brain to react. It starts to produce proteins. The cell should help the body turn out finished antibodies that are the exact shape and form to fit the intruding germ and kill it. It's at this point that the effect of the virus is finally revealed. The virus message then overrides the entire cell system and orders a new product to be made: thousands and thousands of HIV messages in genetic code. These are then carried to the outside wall of the cell where each is wrapped and thrown out of the cell. So infected white cells become factories for more virus, instead of factories to help the body make antibodies.[9]

You can see special electron microscope photographs of hundreds of these viruses appearing as little bulges as they poke out from the cell. Eventually they emerge as little round balls, and the cell dies. Millions of virus particles are released into the bloodstream, each one floating in the blood until it touches another T4 white cell, bursts, injects its message, reprogrammes the cell, and the process continues.

The trouble is that despite all our modern technology it is almost impossible to detect an infected cell. They look identical from the outside until they are dying. The only way we can detect if a cell has been reprogrammed is to kill it, remove the nucleus and examine it. Nor are we able to find the virus easily when it is floating in the bloodstream.

Antibodies don't protect you

The extraordinary thing about the virus is that its outer bag is formed from your own cell membrane. When it came out from the white cell, it was clothed in cell membrane, so its outer feel is just like a human cell. It is true that there are some distinguishing marks on the outside of the virus and the body does produce antibodies. However, when the antibody latches on to one of these lumps on the virus coating, the lump breaks off, leaving the virus intact just as a lizard sheds its tail.[10]

The problem with HIV is *not* that the body cannot produce antibodies against the virus. On the contrary, almost everybody produces antibodies. That is how we test for infection: not by looking for the virus, but by testing for antibodies. The sinister thing is that the virus is *immune* to antibodies. No antibodies have yet been found in a human being that are effective against HIV. That is why a vaccine will be so difficult to find. It is easy to produce antibodies against the virus, but we don't know how to produce one that will prevent infection because we have no natural model from which to work.

New strains of HIV appearing

The other worrying thing about this virus is its ability to alter its shape.[11] Earlier we saw that antibody-producing cells are specific. An antibody against one organism is only rarely effective against another. If an organism changes its outer coating at all, it is back to the drawing board to make a new antibody. HIV can change shape in subtle ways in the same person over the course of a few months, and a person can be infected with several differently shaped viruses at once, possibly with varying abilities to cause disease.[12] Even worse, HIV occasionally changes its shape radically. We are currently seeing new HIV-like viruses emerging every year or two somewhere in the world.[13] There are probably at least four HIV-like viruses already.[14] An increasing number of people are infected with more than one type of HIV. Every time someone is infected, there is a minute chance that radical new changes will occur. As the number of infected people worldwide continues to double each year, so does the risk of new strains emerging. Incidentally, some of our tests for infection are for the earliest virus type found. The others can be missed.

The common cold virus is also unstable. That is why we are always getting colds. I probably have antibodies in my blood now to fifty or one hundred different shaped cold viruses. By the time one of those viruses has infected people between here, North America, Japan, Korea, India, Greece, and back again, its shape has changed so much that I can catch the same cold all over again. That is why we are light years away from a vaccine against the common cold.

The flu virus is also unstable, but less so. We can usually reckon on two or three different viruses causing most flu for a year or so before changing. We spot the new ones, make a vaccine, and give it to people each year. This annual vaccine has never been popular. Why? Because it often gives people a mild dose of the very flu they were hoping not to catch in the first place.

AIDS vaccine could give you AIDS

Even if—and a big if—we could create a new vaccine radically different from any other we have ever made, one that somehow could make the body produce antibodies that latch on to any kind of HIV, whatever its shape, there is the worry at the back of people's minds that it could have some serious side effects.

Vaccination of animals against viruses similar to HIV made the animals ill. Shortages of chimpanzees mean that animal testing will have to be skimped, and that vaccines wlll almost certainly have to be tested first on humans.[15] Even if vaccines did not give people AIDS, there is the possibility that they might get ill more quickly if infected later.[16] Imagine giving ten thousand New York school children the new vaccine. How many years do you think it would take before we could be 100 per cent sure that none of them would ever go on to develop AIDS with the vaccine? The answer is probably five to fifteen years because that is the time scientists now think it can take to develop AIDS. Testing of vaccines requires human guinea pigs. On whom are we going to try it?

There is the possibility that we could make millions of virus particles without damaging messages inside.[17] This should be safe but may not be effective. Damaged virus particles tend to produce a very poor immune response and are usually very poor vaccines. Almost all the effective vaccines we possess depend on a milder form of the virus actually infecting the body. Polio vaccine is an example. But there is no milder form of AIDS that we dare risk giving people.[18]

How vaccine works

Without vaccine	**With vaccine**
virus particles enter nose or lungs	virus particles enter nose or lungs
virus particles enter cells	antibodies ready
reproduce	most virus particles destroyed
increasing number of cells killed	few cells infected
symptoms of flu	mild symptoms
antibodies start to form in 3 days	massive increase in antibodies within 24 hrs
virus numbers start reducing	infection never gets a chance
infection over	

The vaccine gives you the same protection as if you have already had this particular flu a few months before. Your white cells have a memory for life. Response is rapid second time around.

Attempts have been made to take a mild virus used in another vaccine (called 'vaccinia') and change it so the outside looks like HIV but is relatively harmless. This may eventually be our best hope. However, as we have seen, the virus may still turn out to be immune to the antibodies produced. Any vaccine, whether effective or not, will cause all those vaccinated to give 'positive' test results, making testing of blood tranfusions, for example, almost impossible.[19]

So then, in summary, we are a long way from a widely available, effective vaccine. In the meantime you will continue to read of countless spectacular claims. Even if a vaccine existed today that was 100 per cent safe and reasonably effective, it would probably take five years to become widely available at reasonably low cost. When it does come, it will almost certainly be useless at treating those millions already infected.

Hope of drug cure?

Our only other hope lies in a drug that could destroy viruses in the blood. We have none that is effective. For forty years we have searched in vain for a single drug that would work well against a virus without killing the person who takes it. When such a drug appears it will almost certainly cure polio, chickenpox, flu, and a host of other diseases from which our only protection at the moment is vaccination. We will undoubtedly find such a drug one day but it is a long, long way off. How do you kill something that does not breathe, does not need food, does not live, and never dies?

There are four target areas where the virus might be open to attack in the body:

1. Before it touches a cell and its genetic code is injected through the cell wall.
2. When the genetic code has been unravelled inside the cell

and the message is being transferred to the cell brain (nucleus) using a special enzyme called 'reverse transcriptase'.

3. When the cell starts to make new viruses.
4. When the viruses start budding out of the cell wall.

All the newspaper reports of so-called 'AIDS wonder drugs' over the next few months will fall into one of these groups. For example, workers at Hammersmith Hospital in London have recently found that a lack of some chemicals in cell walls seems to make it much easier for the virus to bud out and escape. Could we try adding a chemical to people's diet or find some other way to restore the balance?

Attempts have even been made to flood the bloodstream with small pieces of white cell wall (CD4) so the viruses are unable to touch living T4 white cells. Another method being tried is to inject antibodies ('neutralising') from HIV positive people to give extra protection to people with AIDS.[20]

Others are now looking closely at the virus to try to find any important piece of 'machinery' which is unique to virus production and cannot be found in a normal human cell. Machines in cells are called enzymes.

Enzymes are what are found in biological washing powders. We understand what they do very well. Like antibodies they are very specific indeed and each enzyme is capable of only one thing. Enzymes either split large molecules into two smaller ones—which is how they loosen dirt in clothing—or take two smaller ones and join them together. There is a particular enzyme that reads the genetic code of HIV to form the message that reprogrammes the cell. It is called 'reverse transcriptase'. The body does not usually make it, and only viruses use it. If we could find a way of jamming it effectively *without bad side effects,* we could prevent viruses from reprogramming cells. We are able to jam various other enzymes in the body. For example, aspirin and arthritis drugs jam an enzyme which makes the most painful substance known to man: prostaglandin. This is produced whenever cells are injured in the body. Nerves are irritated by it and fire thousands of electrical impulses which your brain understands as pain. By jamming this enzyme, prostaglandins are reduced and pain is lessened.

Poison for life?

There would be one terrible problem with all such potential drugs. If they can be found, they will have to be taken for life. If some cells in the body are already infected, then a drug preventing entry of new viruses into unaffected cells will need to be taken until every reprogrammemed cell and its descendants are dead—which could take fifteen years or longer. If we stopped the drug after ten years and a single reprogrammed white cell were to be activated to make more virus particles, the disease would start progressing all over again. This applies also to drugs preventing reprogramming, virus manufacture, or budding from the cell.

Almost all drugs have side effects and this particular range of drugs will probably have more than their fair share of them. Zidovudine (AZT), for example, which works by jamming the enzyme reverse transcriptase, is also a poison to the bone marrow of the body which produces all your blood cells. You can die from taking too much Zidovudine for too long, and Zidovudine-resistant strains seem to be developing rapidly.[21] Many people need regular blood transfusions to keep going with the treatment. Every other drug currently being tested has been found to be poisonous to some degree or other. In fact, some are so obviously dangerous that the only way a license can be obtained to give them to human beings at all is because it is on the strictest understanding that all the 'human guinea pigs' are going to die soon anyway from AIDS so a death from the drugs is less serious, even if the hope of cure is remote.

The United States federal government is usually extremely strict on new drugs. Drugs have to be tried on vast numbers of animals for years before they can be tried on humans. The United States federal government has never approved so many half-developed products so quickly, propelled by a ghastly sense of urgency for the million or more United States citizens already infected.[22] The same is likely to happen in the United Kingdom.[23]

So the drugs currently being tried are suitable only for those already affected by AIDS, and while some may be suitable for those who have only become infected, they are completely unsuitable for giving to the whole nation.

However, as doctors are now seeing such a large proportion of those infected go on to develop AIDS, the pressure is growing to try using these drugs on more and more people at a much earlier stage.

Vaccines—a high risk business

Drug companies are pouring billions of dollars into research to find better treatments and much less into vaccines. With a lot less work they can rush through testing and licensing and bring a new drug onto the market.[24] Advertising is unnecessary. Media hype does most of it, and pressure becomes irresistible from patients who are desperate for any hope of cure. Doctors and governments are forced into using drugs which are very expensive—$4,000 per patient—but may hardly work at all and may actually make the patient worse.[25] Of course we need research trials but they need to be carefully regulated. You can spend millions on a treatment for five hundred to one thousand patients, or maybe for the same money get five hundred fulltime health educators on the road into schools, clubs, colleges, factories, and offices, preventing maybe twenty thousand or more extra AIDS deaths a year. New treatments have greatly increased the cost of treating someone with AIDS from diagnosis to death.

Vaccines are a different matter altogether: they are very complex to make and many doubt we will ever be able to make one for AIDS that works and is safe. A long period of investment is required over five to ten years before any drug company that develops a vaccine is likely to earn any money. Even if a company creates an effective vaccine, there is a risk of financial ruin if the vaccine turns out to have serious side effects. In the United States, public liability laws and the vast size of lawsuit claims make drug companies vulnerable to bankruptcy if they market something which turns out to be unsafe.[26]

AIDS is big business and many other organisations stand to gain or lose millions of dollars over what happens. A furious argument over who first discovered the AIDS virus took place between French and American scientists. At stake were world rights to royalties from every blood test for AIDS. After several years the row continues.[27]

Governments need to look at this urgently. No one expects drug companies who operate on behalf of shareholders to go bankrupt in the public interest. They need to be reasonably sure of a return, or if the risks of heavy losses are too large, they need some kind of financial inducement such as low taxation on profits from AIDS vaccines. Failure to address this fundamental issue could set back progress by a decade.

The United Kingdom Wellcome Foundation, which dates back to the yellow fever vaccine developed by Sir Henry Wellcome, is the world leader in vaccine research and production. Currently, millions are being poured into the development of new vaccines—for malaria, for example—but rather less money into AIDS vaccines. On the other hand, a vast investment by Wellcome has produced the world's main anti-AIDS drug, which is selling well.[28] For many drug companies the risks of failure are considered too great to justify a search for an AIDS vaccine. The problems of finding any human volunteers are also considered insurmountable.[29] Companies are waiting for a British government laboratory to come up with a good vaccine they can test. They might then be interested in marketing it.[30]

There are many examples where people may be making money out of AIDS in various ways.[31] Pacific Dunlop (condoms and surgical gloves) profits grew by 31 per cent in six months of 1987 due to the AIDS scare.[32]

Viruses as drugs by the year 2000?

There is a fascinating possibility that by the turn of the century scientists and doctors will be able to programme back to normal any cell that has already been reprogrammed by a virus. Suppose a cell has been taken over by a virus and the book of life is now altered. In the laboratory they painstakingly write a new message and put it into genetic code. Then they (somehow) place the new code into an empty virus bag. The test-tube virus is now allowed to touch a white cell. It enters and releases the new message which programmes back the 'book of life' so it reads normally.

If you are familiar with computers, it is a bit like recreating a corrupt disc. We are a long way from this, not least because most viruses get cells to produce a special chemical called interferon as soon as they have entered, preventing a second virus from entering the same cell, whether a wild one or a test-tube virus.

However, when these tools for tinkering with genetic code of cells in our bodies become available we will begin to see cures for some genetic diseases—maybe even for people with Downs Syndrome, cystic fibrosis, and many others. Perhaps you will one day be able to buy a bottle of hair colour that works permanently. You take it as medicine and the viruses in it reprogramme all your hair-producing cells to produce jet black hair instead of red hair.

Like most major discoveries, it could also turn into a terrible curse: the ultimate in biological warfare. An infectious organism that causes all newborn babies to have no brains, or four legs. A drug that causes children to grow one foot taller by adult life.

AIDS as biological warfare?

Some have suggested that AIDS is the result of a laboratory accident. HIV was made, they say, in a search for new germs for use in wartime and escaped, or was tried out on a few human guinea pigs and spread wildly across the world.

Although it is conceivable that we now possess the means to do this, we know that HIV virus first appeared at least as far back as the early 1970s and possibly as early as the 1950s.[33] Similar viruses are common in some animals in some countries and have probably been around in one form or another for centuries.[34]

Ten years ago we hardly understood anything about viruses. Six years ago we could not even locate the human code for insulin, let alone anything else. It is totally impossible that this virus was first made in the laboratory, although it is possible that it mutated in a laboratory from an animal virus used to infect human cells in a test-tube experiment.

Testing claims for 'wonder drugs'

When you read a newspaper report, take great care. Medical journals are full of papers which contradict others published only a month or two before. This happens because some studies are badly set up or have very few patients in them. If you throw two dice three times and get three sixes, two ones, and a three, you could write a little report saying that you conclude that the dice contain lots of sixes, no twos, and no fours or fives. Everyone would laugh at you because they can pick up the dice and look at them. So what went wrong with your research? You threw the dice too few times to comment and you failed to understand how dice work.

Now if, on the other hand, you threw the dice ten thousand times and half the time they came up with sixes, you might correctly conclude that the pair of dice behave as if they are weighted. If you wrote a newspaper article telling people that all dice from a particular shop are weighted people might believe you—particularly when they hear you threw the dice ten thousand times. You and they would be wrong. How can you generalise about all dice when you tested only two?

You may think these illustrations are an insult to your intelligence, but research workers all over the world make classic blunders every day in the same way. You may not think it possible but it is.

Take the pill for example. A very effective contraceptive—but is it safe? Every now and then there is a large increase in the number of pregnancies, many of which unfortunately are ended by abortion. These usually follow some report or other from somewhere in the world that the pill may cause some rare cancer or problem with blood or whatever.

Even if the reports are true—and they are often contradicted by others published months before or after but *not* reported in the press—there is a vital fact missing. None of the reports points out that to be pregnant carries a risk to life. A small risk, but a risk nonetheless. Abortion also carries a risk. The risk to most women is *far* less from continuing to use the pill than from changing to the notoriously unreliable condom[35] with the possibility of a new unwanted pregnancy.

So then, how do we assess the newspaper scoops on new wonder drugs? Ask yourself what the drug does. Where does it act on our scheme of things earlier in the chapter? What are the risks of taking it and how long do you need to take it? How many patients has it been tried on and how many of them have died? People feel better after taking a Smartie if you tell them it is a wonder drug. This is called the placebo effect. Did these patients know they were being given a wonder drug? If they did, then no wonder they reported feeling better. Your own doctor will be able to advise you on these things. The vast majority of so-called wonder drugs are nothing of the sort, so do not be too disappointed by the negative reaction of your doctor when you show him a press clipping.

When several research papers say the same thing, when each study contains a large number of people with objective results, e.g. numbers still alive after two or three years, then we can start to feel more confident.

Having seen what a virus is, and how the HIV enters and destroys a cell, we can now begin to look at what happens to the body when large numbers of these cells start to die.

3

When the Cells Start to Die

The virus causing AIDS enters the blood and quickly penetrates certain white cells (called 'T4' cells) in the body. As we saw in the last chapter, they programme the white cells after which there is often no trace of the virus at all. This situation lasts for six weeks to nine months or longer. During this time the person is free of symptoms and all current tests are negative.

When infected cells start to die, the first thing that happens is that many people develop a flu-like illness. This may be severe enough to look like glandular fever with swollen glands in the neck and armpits, a feeling of crushing tiredness, high temperature, and night sweats. Some of those white cells are dying, virus is being released, and for the first time the body is working hard to make correct antibodies. At this stage the blood test will usually become positive as it picks up the tell-tale antibodies. This process of converting the blood from negative to positive is called 'sero-conversion'. Most people do not realise what is happening although when they later develop AIDS they look back and remember it clearly. Most people have produced antibodies in about twelve weeks.

Then everything settles down. The person now has a positive test (though not always), and feels completely well. The virus often disappears completely from the blood again.[1] We do not know how many 'body positive' people will go on to the next stage. As we saw in an earlier chapter, at first doctors thought it might only be one in ten, then two or three out of ten. Now it looks as though at least nine out of ten will develop further problems.

Some scientists and doctors are convinced that if we follow up 'body positive' people for long enough—maybe for ten to twenty years—then all or nearly all will die of full-blown AIDS.[2] How long can someone live before some infection triggers production of more virus and death of more white cells?

The next stage begins when the immune system starts to break down. Several glands in the neck and armpits may swell and remain swollen for more than three months without any explanation. This is known as persistent generalised lymphadenopathy (PGL). We do not yet know how many people with PGL will develop further disease.[3]

As the disease progresses, the person develops other conditions related to AIDS. A simple boil or warts may spread all over the body. The mouth may become infected by thrush (thick white coating), or may develop some other problem. Dentists are often the first to be in a position to make the diagnosis.[4] People may develop severe shingles (painful blisters in a band of red skin), or herpes. They may feel overwhelmingly tired all the time, have high temperatures, drenching night sweats, lose more than 10 per cent of their body weight, and have diarrhoea lasting more than a month. No other cause is found and a blood test will usually be positive. This is called an AIDS Related Complex, an AIDS Related Condition, or ARC.

It seems that every person with ARC develops AIDS eventually. You can easily panic reading a list like this because all of us tend to read about diseases and think instantly we've got them. Chronic diarrhoea does not mean you have AIDS. Nor do weight loss, high temperatures, tiredness, and swollen glands.

At the moment there is an epidemic of viral illnesses which cause fevers, tiredness, and other symptoms that last a long time, always go away completely, and have nothing to do with AIDS. See your doctor or go to a clinic for sexually transmitted diseases (STD) if you are unsure.

The final stage is full-blown AIDS. Most of the immune system is intact and the body can deal with most infections, but one or two more unusual infections become almost impossible for the body to get rid of without medical help—usually intensive antibiotics.

These infections are a nightmare for doctors and patients. The desperate struggle is to find the new germ, identify it, and give the right drug in huge doses to kill it.[5] The germ may be hiding deep in a lung requiring a tube (bronchoscope) to be put down the windpipe into the lung to get a sample. The person is sedated for this. It may be hiding in the fluid covering the brain and spinal cord, requiring a needle to be put into the spine (lumbar puncture). It may be hiding in the brain itself. It may hide in the liver or gall-bladder or bowel. It can hide anywhere.

The most common infection is a chest infection. A twenty-three-year-old man walks into his doctor's office with a chest infection not responding to antibiotics. He is flushed and has a high temperature. He has been increasingly short of breath with a dry cough for several weeks. He becomes breathless and has an emergency chest X-ray. The X-ray is strange. No one has seen anything like it before. Could this be AIDS? Samples are taken from the lung. The man is rushed to intensive care and is too ill to ask if he would agree to a blood test. Within two days he is dead. A strange germ is found in his lung: *pneumocysti scarinii*. This is incredibly rare except in AIDS. He may or may not be reported as a statistic to the centre collecting information on AIDS. This is voluntary and doctors are busy. If he had died a day or two earlier, the cause of death would have been thought to be pneumonia. Yet another silent victim, unnoticed and unrecorded. All our statistics may be artificially low, and remember, no test was done for HIV.

He was unlucky. Average life expectancy if you develop your first pneumocystis pneumonia is just over a year, 78% survive the first episode, only 40% survive the second. The average gap between pneumonias is about 6 months.[6] You could live for over three years, or you might be dead in three months. Each new chest infection could be your last. Often people seem only an hour or two from death, then pull around, recover completely, and go home for several months until the next crisis.

We know that eighty-five out of one hundred people with these chest infections are infected with *pneumocystis carinii,* but many are infected with several things at once.

A man is being treated for his second pneumocystis pneumonia. He is really thin now and is developing the hard blue marks in his skin of the Kaposi's sarcoma. He also has a sore mouth because of thrush and boils all over his face. He has a tube in his vein for his high-dose antibiotics. He is feeling ill and tired. Although his chest is improving, one morning he complains of headaches and feeling giddy. He is violently sick and becomes confused later in the day. He gets up in the night and asks for breakfast. He falls over and has to be put back to bed. The following day urgent brain scans are ordered and samples of spinal fluid are taken. Is this meningitis—an infection of the brain surface?

Every test is negative and he rapidly gets worse. He becomes very sleepy and weak and his chest gets worse again. He dies peacefully four or five days later. What caused it? Who knows? A strange infection of his brain? Is HIV directly attacking his brain?[7]

Half of the people with AIDS will develop signs of brain impairment or nerve damage during their illness. In one person out of ten it is the first symptom.[8] HIV itself seems to attack, damage and destroy brain cells of the majority of people with AIDS who survive long enough.[9] The virus is probably carried into the brain by special white cells called macrophages, which then produce more virus there.[10] Brain cells have a texture on their surfaces similar to certain white cells (T4) which enables the virus to latch on and enter.[11] The damage happens gradually and often is not noticed until a significant part of the brain has been destroyed: a brain scan shows a shrunken appearance with enlarged cavities. The signs are threefold: difficulties in thinking, difficulties in coordinating balance and moving, and changes in behaviour. Sometimes the problems are caused by other infections spreading throughout the body, or by tumours, all brought on by AIDS.[12]

A thirty-year-old man is fighting hard to get home again and be independent. He has known about his infection with HIV for over three years, ever since he went to the STD clinic complaining of constant diarrhoea, weight loss, and tiredness.

Having recovered from one chest infection, he is now learning to walk safely without falling over. He is becoming forgetful, cannot remember a telephone number for even two seconds, and is very aware of his shortcomings. With the help of two loyal friends, and our support team of nurses and volunteers, he manages to go home and stay there for a few months. A volunteer rings one day, because he has become gradually more unwell over the last week, is fighting for breath, and has become very frightened. He is readmitted and, despite all therapy, dies a week later.

A sixty-three-year-old man spends all day asleep at home. He has been unwell and has lost weight. He is sent to the emergency room of the hospital. He has been a practising homosexual but has not had sex with anyone for six or seven years. He agrees to an HIV test when all other tests are negative. The test is positive. He is extremely confused, and he becomes incontinent of urine and is catheterised. He lives with a friend who cannot manage him at home. After several weeks, he is transferred to an AIDS hospice unit. Apart from dementia, he develops few other problems and dies peacefully of pneumonia some four months later.

Brain damage affects children as well. In one study, sixteen out of twenty-one children with AIDS developed progressive brain destruction (encephalopathy).[13] But any part of the nervous system can be damaged in adults or children, not just the brain, and AIDS can mimic just about any other disease of nerves.[14] AIDS can develop differently in children. Some children seem able to live with HIV infection for years. Blood tests are often confused by the presence after birth of the mother's own antibodies, and children who later test negative may still carry HIV. If first infected in the womb, the child may regard HIV as part of itself and not react to it.[15]

The majority of people with AIDS develop skin problems which are usually an exaggeration of things common to most people, such as acne and rashes of various kinds. These can develop as part of the pre-AIDS syndrome (ARC).[16] Cold sores and genital herpes may develop, or warts. Athlete's foot in severe forms, ringworm, and thrush are common. Rashes due to food allergy are also common—no one knows why. Hair frequently falls out. Drug rashes often occur, usually due to lifesaving Septrin (co-trimoxazole) used for the *pneumocystis carinii* pneumonia.[17]

Kaposi's sarcoma develops in about a quarter of the people with AIDS: blue or red hard painless patches on the skin, often starting on the face. In the majority of these people it is the first sign of AIDS. Tumours can spread to lymph nodes, gut lining, and lungs where they can be confused with pneumocystis pneumonia. The growths may be caused by a second virus that is allowed to grow more easily if you have AIDS.[18] Treatment consists mainly of chemotherapy and radiotherapy. Because it often affects the face or may be visible elsewhere on the body and is so distinctive, people who develop Kaposi's sarcoma often feel especially vulnerable. In fact people usually live longer if they first develop this tumour than if they first develop a pneumocystis pneumonia.[19] Kaposi's sarcoma is almost unknown in drug users with AIDS, presumably because it is caused by a second virus also found in gay men, which is then activated by HIV.

The other common cancer is a tumour (lymphoma) which develops in the brain or elsewhere in the body.

Almost all people with AIDS have stomach problems from strange infections[20] and cancers caused by AIDS and HIV attacking the gut directly. All three cause food to be poorly digested resulting in diarrhoea and weight loss. Stool samples can be examined or samples can be taken from within the gut using special tubing (endoscopy) to see if there is a second treatable infection in addition to AIDS. AIDS can also seriously affect sight by allowing an infection of the back of the eye (retinitis).[21] This is sometimes amenable to treatment.[22] In addition, the virus can cause damage to other organs of the body such as the heart.[23]

So, now that we have reviewed how the virus attacks cells and causes diseases associated with AIDS, we are in a position to look at some of the ways the virus can enter the human body and how we can prevent it from happening.

Table 1 AIDS Classification (1987)

This classification of HIV disease is now replacing the terms ARC and AIDS.

Group 1: Acute infection—transient illness.
Group 2: No symptoms or signs.
Group 3: Persistent generalised lymphadenopathy.
Group 4:
- a. Constitutional: fever > one month; weight loss > 10 per cent; diarrhoea > one month.
- b. Neurological: encephalopathy, myelopathy or peripheral neuropathy.
- c. Secondary infections:
  - c1. Pneumocystis, cytomegalovirus, toxoplasmosis, etc.
  - c2. Oral hairy leucoplakia, widespread herpes zoster (shingles), salmonella, tuberculosis, oral thrush.
- d. Secondary cancers: Kaposi's sarcoma, non-Hodgkins lymphoma, or primary cerebral lymphoma.
- e. Other conditions.

However, many doctors are now finding it more helpful simply to divide those infected into two groups: HIV well and HIV unwell.

4

How People Become Infected

Different groups of people tend to become infected with HIV for different reasons. Children, drug addicts, sexually active homosexuals, and heterosexual men and women are all developing AIDS in particular ways. Whole family groups are now becoming ill.

How children get infected with HIV

By 1991 there may be at least 10,000–20,000 HIV infected children in the US.[1] A friend of mine cared for his first 'AIDS baby' last week: as a doctor attached to an intensive care unit for newborn babies, he was called to see a baby with a high temperature. He looked for a chest infection and then wondered if the cause was meningitis. Eventually my friend suspected AIDS. His consultant decided a test should be done, not dreaming for an instant it would be positive. Several days later the result came back and it was.

There was an outcry from the staff: a mixture of sadness for the child, anguish over whether to tell the mother who seemed perfectly well but was likely to be the source of her child's infection, and fear of getting the disease from the many needles used in care of tiny babies who are very sick. The child meanwhile had recovered with high doses of antibiotics and the mother had taken the baby home. Both were from abroad and were uncontactable. What is your reaction? (See page 125 for discussion on the ethics of testing without consent.)

1. Infection before birth

Some people used to think pregnancy could shorten the life of someone infected with HIV. Doctors now think the risk of rapid deterioration is not very great.[2]

The baby of a woman who is infected has a 20 to 50 per cent chance of being infected and dying within a year or two (estimates vary). The number of infected babies is rising fast in the United States as the number of infected female drug addicts rises. In New York one in sixty-one newborn babies is born to an infected mother.[3]

2. Infection just after birth

Mother's milk can carry the virus from mother to child. This is an unusual means of infection but is worrying enough for some hospitals in the United Kingdom to discontinue milk banks for sick babies. In fact the risk of getting infected from a milk bank is small because the number of infected mothers is small and probably far outweighed, for the moment, by the advantages to tiny babies of drinking human milk, especially in Africa where sterilising bottles may be difficult.[4]

3. Vaccinations/injections

In Eastern Europe and Africa infection has spread through using the same needles between patients. If there are only a few needles left which are not hopelessly blunt, the temptation is great to immunise a whole clinic with a single needle. Blood from one infected child can spread the disease to others in the group. In some parts of Africa many medicines are injected rather than swallowed. Mothers seem to prefer it. (See 'The African Experience' p. 22.)

4. Transfusions

Unfortunately some children received blood or products made from blood before testing and heat treatments were started in 1985. A terrible tragedy is that over half the people in the United Kingdom who have a severe form of the rare haemophilia bleeding disorder and were given blood products in the mid 1980s are now infected (around twelve hundred people), many of whom are children (around two hundred and forty). Many Romanian children received infected blood.[5]

5. Incest/sexual abuse/child prostitution/early teenage sex/drugs

A thirteen-year-old girl shyly came up to me with a friend after a talk I gave to her class. I had to ask her teacher to leave before she could bring herself to speak. She wanted to know if someone could get infected with HIV through being raped. She was thinking of someone in particular. I had to say yes.

I was talking to a church leader recently who has an eight-year-old boy in his church who is infected. No one knows how. We are going to see an increasing number of these tragedies. In New York, a self-appointed orthodox rabbi fled to Israel after being accused of assaulting one hundred children under the care of his private psychology clinc. Nearly a third of these children are now infected.[6] A child has become infected after sexual abuse by the mother's boyfriend.[7] Five children in Australia have developed AIDS after being sexually abused.[8] Child prostitution is a major worry in London. A professor of paediatrics at a London teaching hospital resigned recently after a child pornography business was discovered (photographs and magazines), although there was never any suggestion that he had acted in anything other than a fully professional way with his patients. The message is that many adult men from a wide variety of backgrounds find children sexually exciting, leading to activities ranging from reading child pornographic magazines to seduction of children to violent molestation. These things have terrible and permanently devastating effects on children and also expose them to the risk of AIDS. Children are also becoming sexually active very young and are not changing their behaviour.[9] Street kids are at high risk. Gonorrhoea and syphilis are common in fourteen- to sixteen-year-olds in New York detention centres.[10]

How drug addicts get infected with HIV

The greatest number of new infections in 1992 is likely to be in the drug addict population of every city and town in both the United Kingdom[11] and the United States. Drug addicts become infected by sharing syringes and needles.[12] A common habit is to rinse the last dregs of drug out of the syringe using your own blood—drawing blood out of your vein and injecting it again. This means the next person injects a lot of virus into the bloodstream if the previous person is infected with HIV. It is far more dangerous than if a doctor pricked himself with a bloody needle. In that case the amount of blood involved would be much less.[13] In Edinburgh, the virus has spread from one addict to infect between one thousand and two thousand other people in eighteen months. In Thailand, fifty thousand drug addicts were infected in two years, with other countries likely to become similarly affected.[14]

The drug addict population is hard to estimate. Addicts do not like to stand up and be counted. Those with children are scared their children will be taken into custody. Others are just shy of any official contact.[15] In the United Kingdom the only ones known about are these who enrol in government programmes to wean them off heroin. Even though this often gives an addict regular drug supplies for life, many are still reluctant to come forward. Recent estimates vary from fifty to one hundred and fifty thousand daily using heroin or similar drugs in the United Kingdom,[16] which includes one to four thousand in Edinburgh and a similar number in Merseyside.[17] In the United States the estimate of drug addicts is thought to be around one to two million.[18] But this may be a gross underestimate. No one knows. AIDS is likely to spread quickly in this group. A growing number are starting to inject drugs other than heroin, such as amphetamines.[19]

The United Kingdom government is willing to give free drugs to addicts to cut out the growing power base of drug bosses. In the United States some say money from drug dealing now exceeds the entire defence budget—in fact it exceeds the entire government's spending. Funds channelled by drug dealers in dishonest ways can destabilise a country; dealers own people, companies, factories, weapons, and they buy votes. Pilot needle-exchange schemes are running in New York City. Volunteers already visit 'shooting galleries' where addicts share needles, giving out bleach and condoms. Methadone treatment centres are expected to increase in number from four thousand to eight thousand just to accommodate the huge rise in the drug addict population. Washington, DC, also has a severe shortage of places for its sixteen thousand addicts. The United Kingdom government is providing free needles at twelve experimental centres in the hope that addicts will be less likely to share them. However, in Italy where needles have been available from chemists for years, over half the addicts are infected. It has been suggested that issuing needles may actually accelerate the growth of drug-abuse.[20] It certainly makes things hard for the police: 'My men are being asked to turn a Nelsonian eye while the addicts uplift their needles,' says one police inspector.[21]

Drug abusers (including alcoholics) have increased risks of becoming infected with HIV in other ways: when they are 'under the influence', judgement is impaired and risks are taken. Safer sex, discretion, and caution are thrown to the wind. So also are safe injecting practices. These people can be hard to educate, not only because they are hard to find and hard to motivate (addicts often have a kind of death wish), but also because, even if they decide to be careful, they soon forget in the rush of the moment.

The third extra risk is that by injecting all kinds of foreign substances—including dirt, germs, and powdered chalk[22]—the immune system is weakened. Addicts frequently come into clinics with huge septic boils, rashes, or strange fevers (septicaemia). They are in no fit state to fight HIV. Infection is more likely and deterioration probably more rapid. An infected addict should be encouraged to stop. It seems that poppers (nitrites) used to increase sexual arousal are also associated with greater risks of infection, probably because they weaken the immune system directly.[23] We are going to hear a lot more about drug addicts and AIDS over the next few years, not least because so many of them are women, and the women then give birth to infected babies or sometimes work as prostitutes. Because of drugs, half the prostitutes in Edinburgh and 13% in New York are infected.[24]

How practising homosexuals get infected with HIV

In the United States of America and the United Kingdom, HIV has spread rapidly through gay communities. Why? There are two reasons. First, it does appear that someone who allows a man to push his penis into his rectum and ejaculate there has a particularly high risk of getting the infection.[25] The lining of the anus is fragile. The lining of the rectum is also likely to bleed during anal intercourse, especially if a pre-sex douche (enema) or a dildo (artificial penis) is used. It is possible that some cells in the rectum have surfaces particularly suited for HIV to latch on to and can become a reservoir for infecting the whole body.

Anal intercourse has always been known to carry a certain health risk: hepatitis B virus is spread easily by this route and many active homosexuals appear to have chronic low-grade infections of various kinds that may then lower their resistance to HIV.

Many people have jumped on these suggestions to reinforce their quite mistaken belief that AIDS is a gay disease. It is part of their mental defences—a desire to turn AIDS into someone else's problem. The fact is that the characteristics of anal sex are not enough to explain what has happened. Anal sex is commonly practised by heterosexuals in the United States and the United Kingdom. Up to one in ten of women questioned report having anal as well as vaginal sex in some surveys.[26] Anal sex alone is not the reason for the spread of HIV. The biggest reason of all has to be found somewhere else, which brings us to the main reason why the gay community is experiencing an epidemic.

If you are an active homosexual, a major predictor of whether you are infected or not has less to do with whether you have anal sex, passive or active, but has to do with the number of different men you have had intercourse with over the last few years.[27] This is only a generalisation. There are people who have become infected after having had sex with only one man. However, in general, the same rule holds true—the greater the numbers, the greater the risk.[28] The trouble is that in the days when only one in one hundred gay men was infected, reducing your numbers of different partners from, say, fifty a year to six a year was likely to reduce your risk of sex with an infected person considerably. But once infection levels rise, the advice breaks down. If every third person you sleep with is likely to be infected,[29] what starts to matter is the number of times a year you have sex with someone who is positive. You might have only three different partners in a year, but if you have sex with one of them for four months you are very likely to get infected. The very promiscuous person in our earlier example, who was sleeping once each with one hundred different men, may in fact have been taking a lower risk: only one episode of infected sex a year compared to the second example of maybe fifty episodes a year. These are reasons why the spread of AIDS will continue even if drastic changes in behaviour occur. The changes need to be even more drastic.[30]

The AIDS epidemic has forced social psychologists to ask some basic questions about human behaviour, questions that may be embarrassing and have been hidden behind closed doors for decades. Questions like: How many people have you had sex with in the last ten years? Do you have sex with more than one person regularly, or are you frequently unfaithful to a regular partner? What sexual techniques do you practise? Have you ever had sex with a man if you are a man, or with a woman if you are a woman? If you are married have you had homosexual sex since marriage? If you consider yourself a homosexual, have you ever had intercourse with the opposite sex?

These questions are extremely hard to get an honest answer to,[31] but are extremely important to enable us to predict how the disease might spread in order to plan effective education. In a clinic for sexually-transmitted diseases some of these questions are asked routinely. The fear of answering can stop some coming for treatment, which is why these clinics have to go out of their way to provide an accepting non-critical atmosphere. Many studies to get further information have been based in these clinics because people have already opened up simply by attending.

The results are fascinating. One of the things that shows up is that sexual behaviour is far more chaotic than many people imagine. Many of us have stereotyped impressions which are miles away from what is actually going on in people's homes, or in the streets.

For example, a United States study has shown that seven out of ten homosexual men have also had sex with women in the last few years.[32] Considering that up to seven out of ten homosexual men in San Francisco (depending on number of partners) are infected with HIV, this is worrying indeed for women in the area. No wonder an increasing number are becoming infected.

Sexual preference sometimes changes with circumstances. A starving man on a desert island will eat strange foods. The reason why there are serious outbreaks of all sexually-transmitted diseases (including AIDS) in prisons is that many men who behave heterosexually outside prison practise homosexuality in prison. I went on two occasions into Wormwood Scrubs to see new prisoners being admitted. All are routinely tested for gonorrhoea and syphilis because if they're not, the diseases could spread throughout the prison in a few months. The same risks for HIV exist in prisons.[33]

Incidentally, in some prisons dominant prisoners will, with the assistance of others, force new prisoners to receive anal sex.[34] This form of initiation brings fear, humiliation, and respect of the boss.[35]

Surveys show that some homosexual men go on to marry and maintain exclusive heterosexual relationships.

However, the most startling fact to emerge from many different studies both in England and in the United States has been the enormous number of different partners some homosexual men used to have in a year. This is in fact no surprise to anyone who has worked in an STD clinic. Dr Fluker, consultant in charge of West London Hospital Martha and Luke Clinics, said in a lecture before he retired[36] that in his experience it was not unusual for some of his homosexual patients to have had three hundred or more different partners in a year—most of whom were met only briefly on one or two occasions.

Over half those attending a London clinic said they had had between six and fifty partners in a year. Many had between fifty-one and one hundred—how do you keep an exact count? Common meeting places are certain well-known public toilets, gay bars, and other known venues.[37] San Francisco officials were so worried about the horrendous risks being taken daily at the bath houses they have all been shut down by law. One senior churchman, himself part of the gay community, told me the reason bath houses had originally been so popular was to ensure that an anonymous pick-up was at least going to be safe. Not safe from AIDS—this was before all that—but safe from violence or murder.

I have attended several post-mortems of people in West London who have been cruelly and savagely mutilated and murdered by an unknown date. Male rape is increasingly common, either by surprise attack in a public place or by a trusted father-figure such as a teacher, youth worker, priest, or stepfather. Sometimes the attacker is alone, sometimes in a group.[38] It is not that gay people are any more violent—you only have to look at the female rape, abduction, and murder figures to see that.

Why the extreme promiscuity by some? The contrast with the heterosexual group is enormous. Very few men will claim to have slept with more than fifteen women in a year. The vast majority claim to have had only one partner in any year.[39] Incidentally that is still unsafe. Each different partner each year is a new risk—even assuming faithfulness by both sides for twelve months. Serial monogamy is very common and is not the answer to AIDS.

When a prominent churchman was appointed as an Episcopalian bishop recently, he was shocked and outraged by what he found in the gay community. What made people do this? What happened to a sense of belonging or relationship? The answer he discovered was that, in 'coming out', many gays had felt able to leave behind conventional restraints such as marriage, home, pregnancy, or anything else.

By deciding to sample 'the fruits of the earth', with no relationship ties, they had found a wonderful new freedom. Even people living together in stable homosexual relationships for years were expected to explore regularly outside that relationship.[40] Public disapproval of gay partnerships also tended to make stable relationships difficult to form and maintain.

In San Francisco, studies have clearly shown that the more partners a homosexual man has had over the last ten years, the more likely he is to be infected. Those with the most partners are the worst affected, with up to 70 per cent testing positive.[41] Remember, though, the people with AIDS that you meet may have had only one or two partners. The best man at the wedding of a friend of mine died a few weeks ago of AIDS. He was an active churchgoer. He had thought seriously about monastic life. He had had only one short homesexual relationship before AIDS was even recognised as a disease and had never been to an STD clinic. You see, just one person can infect one hundred others in a year, some of whom may never have had homosexual sex before and may never do so afterwards.

The other popular misconception is that because many gay men have such a frisky lifestyle, they are uncaring. One of the most impressive things about the Shanti project[42] in San Francisco, or the Terrence Higgins Trust in London, or Body Positive, is the warmth of care, love, and compassion among the volunteers and friends of the person with AIDS.

I think that this is where one of the stereotypes may be true: many gay men have a gentleness and softness that people usually expect to find in women. That is why women make such excellent nurses, mothers, and comforters. Shanti is full of such female characteristics despite the virtual absence of women. The quality of caring is exceptional and is similar in many ways to that which exists in a church like the one I belong to. The paradox is that in my church it is in the context of faithful happy marriages, extended families, positive celibacy, or waiting for the right person. In the gay communities in the past, it has often been in the context of multiple casual sexual encounters.

It is important to understand the reason why. Gay people have felt totally ostracised and rejected by society. Beaten up in alleyways, labelled as perverts, and victims of relentless low-grade discrimination, they have often felt misfits. Rejected by family and former close friends, many have found tremendous security and self-acceptance among others who have been through an identical experienee. The feeling of togetherness is strong. At last they can be themselves without fear of rejection. This fear is often of heterosexual men. Women are usually more tolerant.

This feeling of intense rejection, isolation, loneliness, and vulnerability is then magnified a thousandfold by AIDS. The illness suddenly blows the cover off a quiet homosexual man. Everyone knows he is gay. 'That queer deserves every bit of it,' is on people's lips, even if unsaid. The person may feel so guilty anyway about his lifestyle that he suspects this is what everyone is saying behind his back, or thinks that he deserves it.

This totally false 'gay-plague' label has stuck and reflected on a whole community who have responded with an amazing mobilisation of talent, resources, and kindness to support and surround people with AIDS with love. Victims, as they see it, not of AIDS, but of horrendous prejudices and discrimination.

No wonder the gay community is so sensitive to the hostile attitudes of some parts of the church. Many people in the gay community have seen AIDS as something that has generated openness and an unprecedented care and concern from people who are not gay: 'Things will never be the same again.'[43] However, others have predicted a possible backlash.[44]

Police arrived at a man's house to arrest him for a suspected crime. They were wearing 'space suits' because they were warned he had AIDS (totally unnecessary). Neighbours saw the suits and set fire to his house leaving his family homeless.

Recently a man went into a hospital for an operation. He was tested for AIDS without his knowledge or consent. He was found to be positive and the result was sent to his doctor. He went to his physician's office one day and as he walked in the door, the receptionist, who opens and files all letters from hospitals to the practice, cried out with a gasp, 'Look, it's the man with AIDS.' The man was stunned. That night the man was attacked and his home was burnt to the ground.[45] Why? Just another form of 'queer bashing'. Both these cases happened in London recently.

A few weeks ago a cinema projectionist in England was fired without warning after seventeen years' employment. The reason given was that he was known to be a practising homosexual. He appealed, of course. Since when has a man's sexuality been grounds for dismissal? In the army, yes, but in a civilian job? The industrial tribunal made history. They actually upheld the decision on the grounds that he was gay and would therefore be more likely to develop AIDS.[46] This decision has had devastating implications for every other gay person in any job in the United Kingdom. The decision was overturned by the Court of Appeal.[47] But the fact remains that he was fired, and his appeal to the industrial tribunal was rejected. Do you think he will ever be able to enjoy working there again? His employer has won. Even after winning his second appeal he was entitled to only a few months' wages as compensation. But for what? A devastated life with terrible public exposure of a private lifestyle.

A survey of 321 companies showed that four out of one hundred would sack people with AIDS immediately, and twenty out of one hundred would ask them to resign. So in a quarter of jobs, someone with AIDS will find themselves on the dole. Only sixteen out of one hundred would take disciplinary action against those refusing to work with someone with AIDS.[48]

We have double standards. In our society we say, 'Do what you like,' but if you are caught there is an outcry. 'It's OK to be gay,' the papers say, until a government official or a spy is caught having an affair with another man. 'Disgraceful,' the papers declare. 'He ought to be sacked or put in prison.' The elderly homosexual man is brought to testify under the bright lights. He hangs his head in humiliation. So much for our tolerant society. The same is true of any sexual indiscretion or hint of one. They all become front-page, full-blown scandals.[49] If you cannot grasp even a hint of the emotional devastation wrought on many gay people by our society, you will never remotely understand why the response to AIDS now from the gay community has been so overwhelming in terms of practical care, time, and financial help.

How women get infected with HIV

Women become infected in several ways. Obviously drug abuse puts them at risk. Their main risk in 1990 or 1991 is sleeping with a man who has had sex at some time in the last ten years with another man.[50] Once is enough for him and for her. They will probably never know because the man will never say. Married women all over the country are discovering that their husbands have been having sex secretly with other men for years. The average interval between marriage and the wife discovering her husband's homosexual preferences is between five and fifteen years. The wives usually first discover when full-blown AIDS is diagnosed. This can happen, too, to a church leader's wife.[51]

Women can also become infected from a heterosexual man who has been infected by another woman or who is a drug addict.[52] Very occasionally a woman can catch HIV from nursing her child with AIDS.[53]

Lesbians are one group of people, apart from those who are celibate,[54] where HIV infection is almost unknown. I know of only one case where a lesbian woman has infected another.[55] However, there may be many more infected who are as yet unknown. Lesbians are at risk if they inject drugs and have heterosexual relationships as well.

How heterosexual men become infected with HIV

A heterosexual man becomes infected by sleeping with a woman who injects drugs, by injecting himself, or by sleeping with a woman who has previously had an infected partner.[56] You will never know unless she tells you. Sex on a single occasion with an infected partner can be enough to infect you.

Heterosexual syphilis is increasing in the United States as heterosexuals continue risky lifestyles.[57]

AIDS and the church

Some churchgoers contracted HIV before they became Christians. It can surface after they have begun new lives and are happily married, infecting their wives and possibly their children as well.

Others who regularly attend church lead double lives: a person can pretend to be one thing for an hour or two a week, and probably at work too, while beneath the respectable veneer he has a drug problem or is sleeping around with men or women. The result may be AIDS.

For some today there is no double life. The risky lifestyle is maintained openly in defiance of traditional church teaching, perhaps in a church led by someone with liberal views.

And tragically, a small but increasing number of church members are becoming infected as missionaries in Africa where they are exposed frequently to medical hazards.[58]

5

Questions People Ask

Every day I am asked questions about AIDS, usually the same ones over and over again. Some are based on reasonable fear—of getting the disease from sleeping around, for example. Others are based on unreasonable fear—maybe a fear of going swimming. Here are some common questions and some answers to enable your fears to be reasonable.

Q. How is AIDS caught?

You cannot catch AIDS. You acquire infection with HIV, the virus which after several years can produce the condition we call AIDS. The virus is spread almost entirely through sex and sharing dirty needles. Other routes are extremely rare. Spreading the virus through normal social contact or even through kissing is unknown.

1. Vaginal, oral, or anal sex can transmit the virus from a man to a woman and a woman to a man. Oral (orogenital) or anal sex also transmits in both directions from man to man, and oral sex from woman to woman.[1] In the words of the United States surgeon general: 'Sex may be hazardous to your health.'

2. Other sexually-transmitted diseases will make infection more likely. Wherever sores (which may be hidden and painless) or pus are, there the virus will be in large amounts. These areas are also entry points.

3. Tears, saliva, and urine do contain virus, but almost always in tiny amounts. The amount is greatly increased by eye, mouth, or urine infection. White cells in saliva carry the virus in up to nine out of ten people with AIDS.[2] The virus needs to enter the body to cause infection. Swallowed virus particles are

kept first in the mouth by gum and cheek linings, and do not enter the blood unless you have mouth sores or cracked lips, and in the continuous pipe we call the gut. They are destroyed by stomach acid. They cannot enter the blood once they enter the stomach. Virus particles inside your gut tubing are no more a part of your body than a plastic bead pushed up your nose. (See question on communion cup below.) Urine will not usually contain much virus unless there is a urine infection.

4. All other secretions from the body may contain virus—especially from wounds. The virus cannot enter your body through the skin unless you have a wound, a rash, or some other cracked area on your skin. The most vulnerable place for this is your hands. Gloves are the best protection.

5. If you are going to 'take a risk', a condom will reduce the risk. Condoms do not give you safe sex. It is safer, true, and reduces your risk enormously if properly used. Nonoxynol spermicide also reduces the risk of infection.[3]

6. Injecting drugs with a shared needle is dangerous. Non-injected drugs including poppers may impair judgement and make risks more likely. Poppers may directly damage the immune system, as may other drugs.

7. Safe sex means one thing: for two people who are currently uninfected to enter into an exclusive faithful relationship for life. The trouble is you may never know. If someone wants to sleep with you that badly he or she may never tell you about previous risks.

Safe sex is coming to mean this: virgins at marriage and mutually faithful for life. I suppose almost safe sex is for two people who have had no sexual contact with anyone for at least nine months to both be tested and both be negative before having sex together. Remember though that one or two out of one hundred infectious people never appear positive on testing, and people may be secretly injecting drugs.[4]

Q. Should I take the test?

Remember that it is no good turning up at the STD clinic or your family doctor the day after you have taken a risk. You need to wait at least six weeks, ideally three months, for your blood to have time to become positive if you are infected.[5] During this time you must not be in any further risky situations.[6]

Some people can be infected but produce a negative test result for up to nine months. Very rarely (less than five times out of one hundred) the test never becomes positive. So a negative result may not rule out infection completely.[7]

Sometimes people have a positive test when there is no virus. That is why every test is usually repeated a few weeks later. The test will only tell you if you are infected, not whether you will get ill or die.

Why are you wanting the test? Are you ready for a positive result and all that could mean? Who would you tell? Could you keep it a secret? Remember it could result in a strong reaction against you from people who know. Will you be able to live with that? Are you sure your family doctor will be able to prevent the result from leaking out? It has happened before.[8] Is his receptionist going to know? Is she discreet? A positive result could prevent you from getting a mortgage or life insurance coverage. People should think through these issues first, with the help of a professional. It is easier to change behaviour after having had a positive test result.[9]

Q. Are some types of condom safer than others?

There are hundreds of different brands available, ranging from latex to animal membrane.[10] The ultra-thin/sensitive varieties are most likely to tear although any condom may tear during anal sex.[11] All latex condoms will rot rapidly if oil-based lubricants are used. Condoms should be used with non-oxynol spermicide. Natural membrane condoms may permit virus to pass through more easily.

In summary, if you are taking a risk you need to use a thick latex condom with non-oxynol spermicide. This will reduce your risk enormously if the condom is correctly and carefully used.

Q. Do the results of an HIV antibody test go on my medical record?

In San Francisco you can go to a clinic and get a completely anonymous test done. In the United Kingdom it is more difficult and the result may land in your clinic or hospital records. At the moment the result is not usually sent to anyone outside the hospital.

Q. Can I share pierced earrings?

No. Inserting an earring can cause a tiny amount of bleeding and the earring can accumulate dried debris. Earrings should not be shared. They should be regarded in the same way as needles. Clip-on earrings are safe. Many stores in New York and several in London no longer allow pierced earrings to be tried on. Liberty's of Regent Street have also banned trying on clip-on earrings after an unpleasant scene when a customer noticed a small cut on another customer's ear.[13]

Q. Is a communal bucket and sponge safe for athletes to wash bloody injuries?

The sponge could transmit the virus by rubbing blood from one player into another player's wound. Clean bucket and sponge with antiseptic between players. The virus can survive in water for limited periods.

Q. Are contact sports safe?

You are far more likely to die from a broken neck or be paralysed for life during rough contact sports than catch HIV. For this to happen, blood from an infected player's body would have to be rubbed into a wound on your body. This is extremely unlikely.[14]

If the whole of one team was infected, obviously the risks to members of the other team would be greater, but at present the number of infected athletes must be very small.

Q. Are swimming pools safe?

Swimming pools are safe. Some councils have taken the absurd step of banning all those infected with HIV from using pools.[15] This has produced widespread alarm.

The only way you could possibly catch HIV at a swimming pool would be if someone carrying the virus cut themselves—say on glass at the side of a pool—and left a puddle of blood which you stepped in cutting yourself on the same piece of glass.

In the pool itself the dilutions are so enormous that I am sure that even if you poured ten fresh pints of blood full of virus into the pool, scientists would be hard pushed to find a single blood cell, let alone a virus particle. My wife and I go swimming regularly with our children and we have no intention of stopping.

Q. What about going to the barber?

This is safe as long as disposable razor blades are used—and preferably disposable razors as well. Shaving tends to draw tiny amounts of blood—maybe too small to see. The old cut-throat razor blade could transmit virus from one client to another. For the same reason, razors should never be shared in a household. British government guidelines were sent to 60,000 barbers and hairdressers in September 1987.

Q. What about contact lens solutions and cases?

The bottles of solution may be shared but lens containers may become contaminated by tears. The plastic or glass lens inserted into the eye could help the virus then to enter the body.

Q. Can the virus survive outside the human body?

People used to think that all the HIV particles became severely damaged after only 20 minutes outside the body. We now know this is untrue: an important paper shows that although most virus particles do become damaged after a few hours, a few may survive after three to seven days in dry dust, and over two weeks in water, although only under unusual conditions. In freeze dried Factor VIII, HIV survives undamaged for months, hence the problems for those with haemophilia before heat treatment began in 1985.[16]

Q. How can we disinfect things?

People used to think that a temperature of 56°C for half an hour or so would destroy the virus.[17] This has now been questioned. A recent study shows that some virus may remain infectious for up to three hours at this temperature.[18]

A solution of one part bleach to nine parts of water (10 per cent) will kill all virus in 60 seconds[19] unless there are thick deposits of blood or dirt. These may inactivate the bleach, or require longer for the bleach to work—up to ten minutes.

For some medical purposes 70 per cent isopropyl alcohol kills virus very quickly, as does a 2 per cent solution of glutaraldehyde[20] or betadine (povidone-iodine 7.5 per cent).[21] The virus is *not* destroyed by gamma irradiation or ultraviolet light—both used to sterilise.[22]

Although it is alarming to think that HIV may sometimes remain active outside the body, cases where this has resulted in infection are almost unknown and are confined entirely to puncturing of the skin with blood-covered medical instruments and other accidents.

The general rule still holds true that outside of sex and shared needles, HIV does not spread.

Q. If I scratch myself with a needle, after it has been used to take blood from someone who is infected with HIV, what are my chances of becoming infected?

Probably much less than one in two hundred from one accidental needle stick injury exposure.[23] You are far more likely to get hepatitis B (up to one in five chance) for which you may need a protective injection within the next few hours.

Q. Is it safe to go to the dentist?

Yes. All dentists sterilise their equipment after each consultation. The risk is not to you, the risk is to the dentist. Every time he gives an injection or draws a tooth there is a slight risk that he will puncture his own skin. If the patient is carrying the virus there is a slight possibility the dentist could become infected. This has already happened in New York.[24] For this reason dentists are now using gloves, masks, and glasses when treating people known to be infected.[25] Some dentists are using gloves and masks when treating all their patients.

Q. What about the risk to doctors and nurses?

Doctors are particularly at risk when they take blood. I have accidentally jabbed myself with a needle many times when trying to fill a blood bottle. Needles should never have their sleeves replaced before being disposed of. A third of accidents occur this way.[26] Casualty doctors are in the front-lines when sewing up wounds. Again I have scratched myself with needles several times while stitching injuries—gloves give only partial protection. At risk most of all are surgeons whose hands may be deep inside a patient with a lot of bleeding, sharp needles, and poor visibility. A friend of mine who is an experienced surgeon at a leading London teaching hospital tells me that he frequently tears his gloves during operations. Blood can also spurt from a small artery into the eye. Thirty-four occupational infections have already been reported, but the real numbers must be much greater—not yet detected.[27]

Ideally surgeons would like to know before starting an operation whether the patient is a virus carrier or not so that they can be especially careful during the operation and in cleaning up afterward. At present doctors are usually denied this information for ethical reasons. (See page 127 for further discussion.) As a result a number of surgeons may die over the next decade. At least three surgeons have already died from an infection passed on by patients.[28]

Nurses could become infected by cutting themselves on broken blood bottles. There are very few cases recorded so far of nurses contracting the infection from dirty needles or blood contaminated 'sharps'. One case has occurred where the virus is thought to have entered through cracks in a nurse's hands caused by severe eczema. She was attending a patient with AIDS, without using gloves, and her hands were regularly covered in the patient's secretions.

There are several reports of people who have become infected from blood or secretions coming in contact with their skin—usually on the hands, face, and mouth.[29] It is certain that many such incidents have resulted in infections which have not yet been detected. Some of these reports were of people who had no reason to suspect a risk from their patients and were unaware of any accident until they went to give blood and were found by routine testing to be infected. This is quite different from the situation where a doctor pricks his finger with a needle used on a patient in an AIDS ward. In this situation a report is made out and the doctor is tested. Few such incidents are missed.

In the normal course of nursing or doctoring, the risk of HIV infection is minimal.[30] Care should be taken with needles, and good quality gloves should be worn if there are cuts or abrasions on the hands.[31] It is true that several medical staff in the United Kingdom, and a greater number in the US, are now infected through caring for patients, but this is a tiny number out of the vast numbers involved in looking after these individuals. (See Chapter 7 for further discussions of ethics and risks.)

Q. Can I get HIV infection from a human bite?

Bites can probably pass on the infection, but the risk is almost certainly very low. I have before me a report[32] where a brother infected another brother. It is thought that the first one bit the second and that was the method of transmission. There is a small but variable amount of the virus in saliva which, it has been suggested, entered through the teethmarks of the bite. New York police are now seen regularly wearing bright yellow rubber gloves when arresting gay rights demonstrators. There have been a number of instances where infected people, or people likely to be infected, have deliberately bitten police to frighten them. But the risk from a bite is very low indeed.

Q. Can you get HIV from mosquitoes?

This suggestion is worrying people all over the world[33]—especially in Africa where the number of people infected with HIV is large and people are used to catching another disease, malaria, from the Anopheles mosquito. This was the most common question asked at the big open-air education meetings I spoke at in Uganda in 1988, and also in 1990.

It is almost certain that no one will get HIV from a mosquito.[34] The needle-like mouth of the insect is so fine that white cells carrying the virus cannot be carried in it or on it from one person to another. Scientists have studied outbreaks of AIDS and malaria: malaria is no respecter of age or sex. If you are bitten, you can get malaria. However there are particular age groups that rarely get infected with HIV—older men and women and older children.[35] These people are not immune to

HIV—they simply have never been exposed to the virus. They have often been bitten by mosquitoes and may have developed malaria. Tests on a variety of insects show that HIV cannot multiply inside them.[36] There is a theoretical risk that bed-bugs could transmit the infection, but it has been calculated that a person would have to be bitten about fifteen thousand times by a bug which had just fed on an infected person in order to contract the virus.

Q. What about tattoos or ear piercing?

Both of these procedures can be hazardous unless properly sterilised equipment is used. The hepatitis virus has been spread by these methods in the past. Always go to a reputable establishment.

Q. What about hot wax treatments and electrolysis?

The wax should be properly heated between treatments to kill any virus. The electrolysis needles must be sterilised or discarded. Again, use a reputable establishment. If in doubt, ask what they do to sterilise equipment.

Q. Can you get HIV from acupuncture?

Not if the needles are sterilised or discarded each time. There is currently no legislation to enforce good standards during tatooing, ear piercing, acupuncture, or other things which could transmit HIV. This may change soon.[37]

Q. Is the communion cup safe?

Yes! An Anglican canon in South London remarked to me recently that by the time communion is over, the cup is sometimes full of bits of saliva, saturated bread, and spittle floating in the remains of the wine.[38] He said it had always given him a strange sensation to drink it all, and then to drink all the water used to rinse it, as is the Anglican tradition. He was not the only one to feel uneasy.

Several elderly women in his congregation had recently started returning to their seats after taking the bread only—because of their fear of AIDS.[39] This was in a church with no gay people known to be a part of the congregation, let alone someone actually carrying the virus. The new Anglican guidelines now permit the wafer to be dipped in the wine as a response to the fear.[40] When I visited Uganda recently, I found many churches had abandoned the common cup. After some teaching we shared communion together—a very moving experience as it was the first time for over a year for many.

Fear, fear, fear—threatening to split congregations. But what are the facts?

True—the virus can survive in water for up to 2 weeks under exceptional circumstances.

True—the alcohol content in communion wine is not enough to damage the virus.

True—the virus can sometimes be found in the saliva of an infected patient.

True—the virus particles from one person could be swallowed by another member of the congregation.

BUT the number of virus particles in a sip of wine is likely to be extremely small and you are extremely unlikely to get an HIV infection even if a number of virus particles do enter your mouth. This is because of an amazing protection your body possesses. It is called epithelium or gut lining.

Viruses or bacteria in your mouth are kept out of your blood by a continuous lining of internal skin which lines your tongue, gums, cheeks, back of your mouth, and throat. Swallowed virus enters a continuous pipeline between your mouth and your anus. There is no break in the lining of the pipe. Nothing can enter your bloodstream from inside the pipe (gut, stomach, etc.) without being digested first. This breaks up what you eat into tiny fragments, and then into molecules of protein, fat, and sugar. The first part of the pipe is stretched out into a bag full of deadly acid (the stomach) which kills the virus anyway in a few seconds. Even if the virus was made of steel it could not enter your blood—it would just pass out the other end.

So the communion cup is safe and I will continue to drink from it. We are not going to see a great epidemic of AIDS through church congregations because of the communion cup. It just will not and cannot happen.[41]

Q. Can my children catch HIV from another child at school?

Some schools are now sterilising the mouthpieces of wind instruments, etc. I think that is a courtesy to other children and parents. The main items to watch are the reeds of oboes, bassoons, and clarinets which should be washed and then soaked in a chlorine solution.[42] Playground knocks and scratches are extremely unlikely to spread HIV. To do so, blood from one child would have to be rubbed into the wound of another. (See earlier question on contact sports.) A 'bloodpact' between two children could spread HIV and secondary school children could spread HIV if they are injecting drugs and sharing needles. This is much more common than parents or teachers often realise. My wife and I would be happy for our children to share a class with an infected child. We are not going to see an outbreak of AIDS spread by school children—except through teenagers injecting drugs or sleeping around.

Q. Can I get HIV from a discarded condom?

The first time many young people ever see a condom is in the street. There it is lying in the gutter, chucked out of a car window the previous night. There is a small but growing risk that the semen it contains is full of virus. It should be picked up with tissue, gloves, spade, or trowel and discarded carefully.

Q. Can I get HIV from being raped?

Yes, it is possible. The risk can be higher because the violence used can make abrasions and bleeding more likely, creating entry points for the virus.

Q. Is it safe to have blood transfusions?

Routine testing of all blood has been carried out to detect HIV since 1985 in the United Kingdom. Unfortunately a number of people were already infected by this time from transfusions. From 1985 to the end of 1986, sixty-four pints of infected blood were detected and thrown away. The risk is now very low.

However, the test does not pick up, for example, the man who gives blood five weeks after sleeping with an infected prostitute while on a business trip abroad. The test can take up to nine months to become positive during which time a donor could give lots of infected blood to the Red Cross. In some cases it never becomes positive even though the person is dying of AIDS. This is because some people never produce antibodies, and others are infected with new viruses not easily detected by the test.[43] At the moment the risk is very low because gay men, drug addicts, and other people who might have been exposed to HIV have been deliberately asked to stop giving blood, and almost all have ceased to do so. However, as the number of infected people in the general population rises, the numbers of infected units that pass through undetected will rise.

If I were about to have a major operation, I would ask for as few units of blood to be used as possible. Blood is not so essential as many people sometimes think. We have some excellent blood substitutes now which can replace the first two or three pints of blood lost unless you started off very anaemic. In the United States there are large numbers of Jehovah's Witnesses who refuse blood transfusions for religious reasons. Few die, however. Major surgery without the use of blood transfusions is now a well practised art in the United States.

It is sometimes possible to arrange to give your own blood which can be stored before your planned operation.[44] This makes you slightly anaemic, forcing your body to make a lot more blood cells.

By the time your operation takes place, your blood is normal again and two or three units of blood are ready for you in the blood bank. The shelf-life of stored fresh blood is only thirty-five days, which is one reason why not many hospitals yet offer this facility.[45] The other reason is cost.

As soon as we have a widely available blood test for the virus itself, not the antibodies to it, we will be almost 100 per cent safe.

Try to avoid having a blood transfusion outside Europe, North America, Australia, or other countries where medical facilities are good. Many other countries have inadequate facilities for testing, although the situation is changing rapidly. (See advice for travellers pp. 183–191.)

For a long time, people too embarrassed to go to a sex disease clinic for a test for HIV antibodies, have been going along to give blood. They know that all blood is tested there. This happened a lot in England until the Blood Transfusion Service woke up to what was happening and tried to stop it. It is terribly dangerous: someone infected last week who goes to give blood gives infected blood expecting it will be detected but it isn't. The test will not be positive for weeks. The blood slips through and is used in a hospital.[46]

This is still going on. Recently, a doctor friend of mine told me that he had heard of a group of friends who trooped down to the Red Cross hoping to get a secret test. They had all been at risk. They all gave blood. Some of that blood may get through and infect a patient.[47]

More than a thousand people in England may die as a result of infected blood or blood products.[48] The government should probably have taken precautions earlier when it was first alerted to the dangers of importing blood products from the United States. They have now agreed that all those infected as a result of this treatment should receive automatic compensation. For those having to cope with chronic bleeding problems due to haemophilia, the knowledge they may now develop AIDS is an even more terrible curse.

Q. Can I get HIV by giving blood?

Not at all. The Red Cross is now short of supplies because many people are afraid of infection and are staying away.[49] But there is no danger at all in giving blood. All the needles used are sterile. There is no risk to you at all.

Q. How do scientists figure out the numbers of people infected from those who already have AIDS?

The rule of thumb at the moment seems to be born out by all the data (see Chapter 1):

- one person with full-blown AIDS
- five to ten people with early disease (ARC or HIV unwell)
- twenty to one hundred people infected, mostly feeling well at the moment

This will change as the disease spreads. For instance, in drug addict communities, one person can infect another one thousand in a few months producing say:

- one person with full-blown AIDS
- one hundred people with early disease
- one to two thousand people infected

Outside the drug user and gay communities, the rate of spread seems to be slower in the West. This could produce:

- one person with AIDS
- five people with early disease
- twenty total infected

This effect could also be produced if the interval is shorter than usual between infection and disease. Therefore the rule of thumb will alter according to the rates of spread in particular groups, the numbers in each group, and the speed at which infected people develop the disease.

Q. Is it safe to kiss someone on the lips?

Yes. The risk of infection from a dry kiss is almost zero, and since the number of infected people in the general population is low, the risk of catching HIV from kissing a girlfriend or boyfriend on the lips must be absolutely minute. A 'French kiss' where tongue and saliva enters another person's mouth carries a higher risk, especially if one person has sores in the mouth, cracked lips, or bleeding gums. However, we have never yet seen a case of 'mouth to mouth' spread.

Q. Can I get HIV from a toilet seat?

No. Obviously a woman who is positive should be careful when menstruating not to leave blood on the toilet and to dispose of tampons or sanitary napkins carefully. Genital contact by another user could result in infection, but the risk is very low. There are no reports yet that the infection has been caught by this means. Despite the myths and statements by doctors, gonorrhoea can be caught from clothing and towels in a similar way. In fact this used to one of the commonest causes of a sore vagina in little girls.[50]

Q. Can I get HIV from sharing a toothbrush?

This is theoretically possible, but we have never seen infection by this route despite careful studies of many families where one person is infected. Brushing causes tiny amounts of bleeding from the gums so a toothbrush should be used by only one person. Likewise, articles such as towels or razors (even electric razors) should not be shared.

Q. Can I get AIDS from the skin of an AIDS patient?

If the patient has weeping boils or other skin problems causing the skin to crack, bleed, or produce secretions, then care should be taken. The secretions may be full of virus. Remember, however, that virus on your own hands is not going to infect you unless there are breaks in your own skin. Hands are especially vulnerable so cover cuts with waterproof bandages and if in doubt, use gloves. Several cases of infection have occurred following heavy contamination of broken skin by blood or secretions. Blood on the face of an infected person with acne or a skin rash has been known to transmit the virus.[51]

Q. Am I more likely to get HIV from an infected person if my hands are cut or sore?

People with eczema should be especially careful to wear gloves when likely to come into contact with secretions from someone with AIDS. The thousands of tiny cracks and itchy blisters are entry places for the virus. Cuts should be covered with a waterproof bandage. Gloves should be worn by all people whenever handling anything covered with secretions or when lifting or turning a person in bed.[52] Obviously gloves are *not* necessary for normal social contact, handling of crockery, or unsoiled clothing.

Q. Can I get HIV from mouth-to-mouth resuscitation?

The same principles apply as for French kissing or communion. I once found a man who had collapsed three minutes previously on the pavement outside Liverpool Street Station in London. I gave him mouth-to-mouth resuscitation for twenty-five minutes until the ambulance arrived. By the end I was covered with his saliva. It was over my face, in my eyes, in my mouth, and in my lungs. Every time I lifted my mouth after giving a breath he spluttered back at me.

You can reduce this risk enormously by covering the mouth with a handkerchief and breathing through it. Hospitals and ambulances carry a special tube connecting your mouth to the dying person. It has a valve preventing air and secretions blowing back in your face. Many police cars now carry these too. They should be standard issue but since they make resuscitation more difficult[53] it probably would not make sense to use one unless you were already familiar with it.

That man walked out of the hospital despite it taking forty-five minutes from his heart stopping to his arrival in the emergency room. Mouth-to-mouth resuscitation saves lives, and if you do not do it because you are afraid of getting infected, you may have to live with your conscience for the rest of your life. The good Samaritan was the one who took the risk of being mugged or robbed to stop and help a dying man lying in the road.

For a man in the street, the risk of the other person carrying the virus is currently low. The risk of catching the virus would be more for someone who knew that the person who had collapsed was positive, had AIDS, was a drug addict, or was known to be a homosexual.

Q. Can you pick up any other infections from someone with AIDS?

Yes. There are two possible hazards: the first is tuberculosis (TB) which can often develop rapidly in someone with damaged natural immunity,[54] and the cytomegalovirus infection.

People with AIDS are one hundred times more likely to have TB than the average person although the kind of TB they have is often less infectious to others.[55] If someone walks into a hospital and has widespread TB, one of the first questions doctors ask now is: Does this person have AIDS?[56] In healthy people tuberculosis is now easily treated.

The other hazard, the cytomegalovirus infection, is very common and usually quite harmless but can be crippling to someone with AIDS.[57] Many people are carrying antibodies to cytomegalovirus due to normal exposure.[58] However, the virus can infect babies in the womb with serious consequences. For this reason some have suggested that no one who is pregnant or could be pregnant should look after someone who has AIDS. But, in fact, the risk of contracting cytomegalovirus from an AIDS patient is still low.

Apart from these, the risks are entirely the other way around, as the simple cough or cold a well person has could make someone with AIDS seriously ill.

Q. What are the main differences between the treatment of people with AIDS in San Francisco and in London?

The differences are extraordinary. In England someone with AIDS spends an average of eighty-six days in a hospital from diagnosis to death, compared with eighteen days in the USA.[59] The average length of each stay on the ward at one hospital in London was seventeen days,[60] whereas when I visited San Francisco General, the average stay had just dropped from eleven to eight days.[61] In London 15–20 per cent of patients will be in hospital at any time compared with 10% in San Francisco.

In some units in London almost every person with a chest infection has a routine bronchoscopy which involves putting a tube with a miniature camera down someone's windpipe when they are already finding it hard to breathe. Often the result of the procedure is a collapsed lung and further procedures to inflate it again. In San Francisco, the strange pneumocystis pneumonia is diagnosed eight times out of ten without bronchoscopy.[62]

Intensive treatment is started and the person is often home in three days while attending the clinic each day for the remainder of treatment. Our community nursing and doctoring for other illnesses are far superior to that generally available in the United States so these differences are all the more remarkable.

Part of the reason is experience: when you are seeing your two thousandth case of pneumocystis pneumonia you start to get very good at diagnosing and treating it. When your one hundredth patient gets stuck on the ward because of increasing dementia, you become far swifter at getting people home before it happens. You also become far more realistic (or pessimistic) about what a prolonged hospital stay will achieve.

But, you may say, why can't British hospitals learn from those on the other side of the Atlantic? Each country usually likes to develop its own method of working. It is a pity that we seem to be missing out on some opportunities to skip four or five years of that learning process. Research in one country must be repeated in another a few years later it seems, and all the while people may suffer unnecessary extra tests and procedures.

Q. What is the importance of a 'doubling time'?

The doubling time is the time it takes for the number of those with AIDS or early infection to double. It used to be six months in many countries first experiencing the disease but is now averaging eighteen months to two years in the UK.

A story is told of a famous chieftain who was agreeing the price of a piece of land: he had a chessboard in front of him with sixty-four squares. He said his price was a grain of wheat on the first square, two on the second, four on the third, eight on the fourth, and so on. The deal was agreed. What the other man did not realise was that by the time he got to square sixty-four, all the grains of wheat in the entire world would not be enough! In around ten doublings you reach one thousand, but by twenty doublings you reach nearly a million. By thirty doublings the number is impossible to even imagine.

A doubling time of six months to a year means it only takes a generation to multiply current numbers by billions. But current numbers infected worldwide are already reckoned as millions.

Q. Could we all be wiped out by AIDS?

No. The spread is likely to slow down as many of the people with multiple partners and drug addicts become infected.[63] The length of time for the number of new cases to double is getting longer in most countries. At the start of an epidemic the doubling time is often six months. After a few years it usually lengthens to more than a year. This is still very serious but at least it shows some sign of hope. The United States took nine months to double from thirty-five hundred to seven thousand cases, eleven months to double from seven thousand to fourteen thousand, and thirteen months to double from fourteen thousand to twenty-eight thousand by December 1986.[64] In Africa, other factors are encouraging the spread in ways we do not understand. Outside Africa the spread throughout the general population will continue, but almost certainly more slowly. Eventually there will be a cure (although conceivably not for ten to twenty years). The only way the whole of mankind might die would be if this highly adaptable, unstable virus were to change its method of transmission. Other similar viruses can be spread through droplets, coughing, and sneezing. We really do not understand fully why this does not happen with AIDS. We are all hoping this will never happen in the future, but it could, and the more people who are infected each year, the greater the chance of such a mutation. If it happened, the whole of mankind could be destroyed rapidly unless we found a cure in time.

Q. Why not test everyone and separate infected from uninfected people?

I am horrified when people ask me this question. This is a recipe for concentration camps. Also it will not work: many infected people will be missed due to the test not becoming positive for up to nine months after infection. Many who think they are positive will disappear and go underground. The days when any country could close its borders are over. Millions of people travel to other countries each year, many illegally. Someone would have to enter quarantine after being abroad for twelve hours because that is long enough to share a needle or have sex. Quarantine would be for up to nine months. During this time the person would have to be kept in solitary confinement in a prison cell so there could be no possibility of sexual intercourse or sharing needles. What would happen to business trips? No tourist could travel without being in a 'sex-free' prison for up to nine months first. What are you suggesting? An iron curtain even more effective and destructive than was the one in the East? Husbands and wives separated on one side or the other? Children never able to see an aunt or an uncle except in a room with a television camera?

Even if the epidemic is controlled in one country, if all neighbouring countries have rapidly increasing problems HIV will find its way in. That is why even if I agreed with the concentration camp idea—and I find it utterly repulsive—I would think it stupid to try it. The answer has to be a worldwide answer. The only alternative is to close all borders, airports, and sea ports and blow up any ship, pleasure boat, or plane that approaches the coast.

Q. If I am positive—or think I might be—how can I best keep well?

First stop risking further exposure. If you are infected, the number of damaged cells so far may be small. Do not increase that by infecting more cells with virus. Secondly, any further diseases may trigger release of more virus into your blood. All infections should be avoided, where possible, whether sexually transmitted or not. Adopt a healthy diet with plenty of rest and exercise. Stop abusing drugs of any kind—even alcohol. Nitrites or poppers may accelerate development of Kaposi's sarcoma and should be avoided.[65]

Q. What is the simple answer to AIDS?

The simple answer to AIDS is, in the words of a doctor from Northern Ireland, an 'epidemic of faithfulness'. Only an epidemic of faithfulness can stop the epidemic of AIDS—together with taking care over dirty needles.

All these questions are important. However, the biggest question in my mind is this: Are condoms really as safe as everyone seems to think they are? Is the emphasis on condoms for safer sex simply because we can't think of anything better to say—or is it really grounded in fact? If it is safer, how much safer is it?

6

Condoms are Unsafe

Whenever I talk to young people about AIDS I find the same thing: they think that using a condom will prevent them from getting HIV. The truth is that it may reduce the risk, but I wouldn't trust my life to a condom.[1]

Condoms are unreliable. If one hundred couples use condoms, up to fifteen of them could be in clinics *each year* asking for abortions.[2]

When taken out of the packet, holes were found in up to thirty-two out of one hundred condoms of the least reliable makes.[3] These holes are defects. The British Standards Institute actually permits three out of one hundred to have holes in them when they leave the factory.[4] In the US, government standards are much higher, tolerating only four condoms out of every thousand to have leaks. But even with this high standard, condom users still experience a failure rate of 5 to 15 per cent, which is the percentage rate of women who have an unwanted pregnancy while using this method of birth control over one year's time.[5] No wonder so many women get pregnant!

A leading medical journal puts the failure rate much higher at 13–15 per cent per year.[6] A spokesman from the London Rubber Company (Durex) admitted that if incorrectly used, the failure rate of condoms could be anything from 25 per cent up to 100 percent; and there are real problems with teaching people how to use them—not least because of illiteracy. Problems of illiteracy are so bad in the United States (one in five adults) that the army is printing manuals in cartoon form. In the United Kingdom, Durex instructions now contain illustrations for the one in ten who cannot read.

The condom is the least reliable contraceptive in wide use—it's as bad as the diaphragm or cap with spermicide. The only thing less reliable is the sponge (up to 25 per cent pregnant each year).[7] Many violently disagree. They say it is a superb contraceptive, it is *people* who are unreliable: they put it on too late or inside out, tear it, forget it, let it fall off. They say people are unreliable but the condom is reliable, if properly used.[8]

Recently there was an outcry about how dangerous three-wheeled invalid vehicles were. 'Unsafe' people said. No one went on TV to say that the vehicles were perfectly safe, it's just that people need to be careful when driving them when going round corners. On the contrary, I think most people saw that an average driver could very easily have an accident through no fault of his own. It is easy to have an accident with a condom. Condoms are unreliable compared to, for example, the pill. That is why the pill is so popular—not just because it is a more pleasant method.

Things are worse than they appear from the pregnancy rates. Out of 100 couples, 10 will have great difficulty in conceiving anyway. Five will probably never be able to conceive for various reasons, including previous infections with sexually-transmitted diseases.

After four months of trying to conceive, only about half of an average group of women will succeed in becoming pregnant. If they used a perfectly safe method two out of three times that they had intercourse, it would take a year for half to become pregnant. If they used the method for ten out of twelve months of the year, then twenty-five out of one hundred could be expected to get pregnant in a year. If they had unprotected sex for one month a year and used the method for eleven months, then it could be expected that over twelve would become pregnant in a year.

What this means is that if condoms produce a failure rate of around twelve in one hundred per year, then they must be leaking often. It is about the same thing as having intercourse for a whole month without any protection at all but taking the pill the rest of the year. Somehow or other secretions from a man and a woman are very frequently meeting each other.

Think about it: a woman can only become pregnant on three days a month—while ovulating and shortly afterward. After a single accident with a condom there is only a one in ten or so chance of it being a fertile day anyway. Even if it were, pregnancy may not follow. However, it is possible to catch HIV infection every day of the month. An increasing number of people have become pregnant recently because they switched from a more reliable contraceptive to the condom because of AIDS.[9]

If up to fifteen couples each year are actually managing to conceive despite condom use, there must be frequent accidents—probably one time out of twelve, from the figures above. If you are having sex regularly with an infected person, it is like throwing dice. Every time you throw a twelve is how often the condom has let you down. Would you trust your life to a condom?[10] Remember that one episode of unprotected sex can be enough to infect you. Over the next few years there will be a growing number of angry men and women who have become infected, despite their using a condom, having thought they were safe.[11]

A recent report has been published on some couples using condoms where only one partner is positive.[12] Up to a quarter of the partners became infected with HIV in only one to three years, despite use of the condom. Others may say these people were careless. All I am saying is that I agree with the Family Planning Association. If correctly used, the condom can be a reliable contraceptive and will almost certainly reduce your risk of getting AIDS, but the reports show that it is hard to use safely. In fact a Danish study of condoms shows that condoms have a failure rate of 5 per cent. If the risk of HIV infection with infected partners is 1 per cent, then someone having sex three times a week will have a 3 per cent chance of infection in one year and 21 per cent in three years despite regular use of a condom.[13]

Another study of partners using condoms suggests that the risk of catching HIV is reduced by 85 per cent.[14] That sounds excellent but it is not. If you persist in sleeping regularly with someone who is positive or with numbers of unknown people who are possibly positive, then eventually, condom or no condom, you may get AIDS. All the Terrence Higgins Trust literature clearly states that vaginal or anal sex using a condom is not a low risk or no risk activity. It carries a medium risk at best.[15] Dr Norman Hearst and Dr Stephen Hulley (Centre for AIDS Prevention Studies in San Francisco) estimated recently that even with condom use an uninfected partner had a one in eleven chance of becoming infected after five hundred sexual contacts.

Condom manufacturers' literature states that condoms are designed for vaginal sex only and are not suitable for protection from AIDS transmission by the anal route. Particularly hazardous is the use of oil-based lubricants as these rot the rubber in minutes.

What is safe sex?

So what is the correct health message? It is that condoms do not make sex safe, they simply make it safer. Safe sex is sex between two partners who are not infected. This means a lifelong, faithful partnership between two people who were virgins and who now remain faithful to each other for life and do not inject drugs. If you are going to have sex in an unsafe situation you are crazy indeed not to use a condom, and you must use it very carefully every single time, preferably with non-oxynol spermicide. But don't kid yourself that you will never get AIDS.

We do not know what the risk is from a single sexual contact with someone who is positive. It certainly depends on many other factors such as whether either partner also has gonorrhoea or syphilis. Any sores will be full of white cells and virus. It seems people are most infectious for the first 12-15 weeks after infection with HIV, and then years later when beginning to feel unwell again. Some individuals may be more susceptible than others. It seems that the risk from a single accident with a condom or a single unprotected contact is small, but some have become infected this way.[16]

Medical advice on using a condom more safely

A condom is tightly rolled up. Make sure it is the right way around. It will only unroll one way. If you make love in the dark you may need to turn the light on. The teat at the end is there to collect all semen and fluids from the man. This needs to be squeezed empty of air or the condom may leak. With one hand holding the teat, the other is used to gently roll the condom over the entire length of the erect penis. This must happen as soon as the man is aroused[17] for two reasons: first a small amount of fluid emerges from the end of the penis during arousal as part of the body's natural lubrication before the man enters the woman. This can be full of virus. Secondly, a woman produces a lot of secretions during arousal for lubrication. These may also contain virus if a woman is infected.[18] The early use of the condom is to keep any genital contact separate from the start.

Wear and tear

A woman usually takes longer than a man to become fully aroused and will usually find things more satisfying if there is continuing caressing before her partner enters her. During this period a condom may unroll partly or fall off altogether. It may also suffer general wear and tear. It can snag on a woman's jewellery or on her fingernails. This can happen if, as advocates of condoms suggest, the woman helps the man put on the condom as part of lovemaking. Damage is usually obvious early on. The real danger time can be when a woman helps her partner come inside her. Fingernails and jewellery can cause a minute tear in the condom which enlarges during intercourse. The result is discovered on withdrawal. Non-oxynol-containing spermicide pessaries should be used for extra safety as they can destroy some of the virus (see pp. 88, 89, 116).

Rapid exit

Withdrawal must be prompt for two reasons: first there is a small risk of semen leakage along the shaft of the penis, especially if the teat was full of air. Secondly, as soon as a man has reached climax, the penis starts to soften and what was a tight fit becomes a very loose fit. Condoms can easily leak or slip off inside a woman. The condom end must be held gently as the man withdraws.

Most people dislike using condoms

A huge campaign is being carried out to try and make the condom more acceptable. When used carefully as above there is no doubt in most couples' minds that it is disruptive and they dislike it: it is a real turn-off. What's romantic about a condom?[19] After all, that is one reason why people stopped using condoms when the pill came along. The other was appalling unreliability and constant fear of pregnancy. It was the pill, not the condom, that brought about the so-called sexual revolution of the 1960s.

1. To put it on carefully takes precious seconds out of a continuing experience. Some men find that by the time they have got it on so they are happy it is comfortable (may need a couple of tries), their erection has disappeared. A woman is left hanging around and rapidly loses her momentum. Trying to find where you put one, opening the packet, and getting it on correctly can be a joke, but it is disruptive.
2. Making sure it does not roll off can cause tension in the pre-intercourse stage of lovemaking.
3. Checking it is still intact immediately before entry causes further delay.
4. Many men say that the layer of rubber reduces what they can feel[20] (although some who tend to ejaculate too early may find that an advantage). Many women dislike the thought of a piece of rubber in such a personal area.
5. For many couples a central part of their celebration of oneness is to be lying together, with the man inside, immediately after both are satisfied. Many people enjoy being able to 'cool off' in each other's arms like this. Correct condom use requires the man to withdraw immediately. Some see it as a rather abrupt and savage end to a marvellous experience.
6. Some find disposing of the used condom rather revolting.

The best method is to tie it up carefully, wrap it up in toilet paper, and flush it away.

In addition there is another vital factor: the very fact that a condom is being used, other than merely to provide some protection against pregnancy, implies slight anxiety about whether a partner is infected. This can cause tension.

Are people using condoms more?

Homosexual men are using condoms more than they used to. This is not surprising since their chances of sleeping with an infected person may now be up to one in three[21] in the United Kingdom or one in two or greater in parts of the United States. However, there is no condom which reliably withstands the rigours of anal intercourse. Young heterosexual people of both sexes were recently interviewed and many said that they were now intending to use a condom as a result of the government campaign. When a similar large group was interviewed about four months later it showed that very few had actually started doing so, who were not before. In other words, the campaign stirred lots of good intentions but no action. In fact over the period in question the number of new cases of gonorrhoea rose in heterosexuals although it fell in homosexuals. So the number of partners was just as high as before except in the homosexual group who were panicked into more restrained behaviour.

More recently a new survey has suggested that UK condom use may be greater than the pill, particularly by young people. People are constantly trying to invent new ways to promote condoms. One company is giving condoms away with every pair of jeans.[22] It is extremely difficult for a woman who has no boyfriend at the moment to buy a packet of condoms and keep one in her handbag. When she goes out for the evening it is hard for her to take a condom. In doing so she is admitting that she might have sex with someone tonight.[23] Many women feel carrying a condom makes them look promiscuous, when they feel they are not. A further major problem is when to produce it. A romantic evening is turning rapidly into something more. Are you going to show you don't trust the other person by reaching for a condom? Will the other person take offence at you implying that he or she has been sleeping around? Insisting on a condom may take a lot of self-confidence and courage on the part of the woman.[24] Female condoms may be easier.[25]

How to minimize the disruption

Be prepared. Talk it through with your partner. Practice! But there is a better way: change your lifestyle. So many pamphlets tell us how wonderful 'safe sex' is. They say how fulfilling and lovely it is just to rub bodies together and have a cuddle. They describe a vast number of other things people can do to have sex safely together. That is not what I call sex—it is a mockery of what was intended and created for us to enjoy. The pamphlets condemn people to a lifetime of nonsense. *'A hundred and one ways to have fun with a condom.'* How lovely. How stupid when the alternative is so simple.

The choice is so obvious and clear. After the Chernobyl disaster in Russia all the animals started to die in farms around the nuclear reactor. Imagine a booklet entitled, *'A hundred and one uses for a dead cow.'* How marvellous. Why not just move three hundred miles to an unaffected area?

Find someone you love and trust—someone who is not infected at the moment—and will remain faithful to you for life and to whom you will remain faithful. Then you can enjoy unlimited, anxiety-free sex. (Advice to spouse of infected partner p. 116.)

Free love

You may reject this. Your philosophy is that if people want to they can sleep together without any great relationship or strings attached. 'We live in a free world and people should be free to do what they like.' Maybe you feel that ultimately you want to be married but you want to have fun now. Friends of mine are afraid that their relationships will become tame and boring if they get married. 'A piece of paper won't make me love her any more.'

As a doctor and as a church leader, I am constantly seeing the casualties of this, and they are usually women. Life is unfair. Somehow it is always the woman who comes off worse: she is the one who becomes pregnant and her risk of catching HIV is probably greater than the man's risk from her. She suffers the chronic pain of pelvic inflammatory disease and cervical cancer. And the woman is often the one who is most devastated when a relationship breaks up.

Free love is fine until your lover leaves you at forty-three years of age, and you still have had no children because he would have walked out. A whole generation of people are growing older. Pensioners of tomorrow with no wives, no husbands, no children, no family—only a few casual relationships and old memories. No wonder many are deciding that enough is enough: the right person has not come along so they are staying single and celibate, yet forming long-lasting, warm, caring friendships. Someone was saying in a newspaper article the other day how exciting it was to commit adultery. She was saying there was nothing wrong in it. There were some angry letters. One woman said that adultery was wrong for lots of reasons: for her it had meant an elaborate web of cheating, deceits, small lies, and big lies. The total betrayal of the trust of another. No wonder it causes such terrible bitterness and hurt. Adultery wrecks marriages and damages children. This is not the best plan for human relationships.

Women leading the way

On a recent TV programme[26] a young audience was voting on love, sex, condoms, and marriage. Huge differences emerged between the boys and the girls. Some boys wanted to 'score' with as many girls as possible. Their reputations and image depended on sleeping with every girl they went out with. Many girls were disgusted. They wanted commitment, friendship, companionship, security—and then they would give themselves in other ways.

Marriage has never been so popular, and the girls are leading the way. It is the girls who are worried about AIDS; many boys could not care less. It is the girls who worry about getting pregnant or being let down. I believe that part of the next education phase needs to be to teenage girls and young women, many of whom need little convincing about the desirability of being in a warm, loving, caring, exclusive relationship. This strategy should be designed to give them moral support when under pressure, not to 'sell themselves cheap'.

It is strange that many men want easy women to have fun with, but deep down prefer by far the thought of marrying a virgin.[27] We need to cultivate a new age where romance is in, self-respect is in, faithfulness is in, marriage is in. I don't think it's clever to sleep around or get divorced.

The people I admire are those who work at relationships, who are good at relationships, who have good happy marriages, who can handle things. What's so smart about walking out on every problem? I respect and admire, too, those people who have made a positive decision—for whatever reason—to remain single and celibate.

Advice to someone married to a 'positive' spouse

You may be afraid you or your spouse are already positive. You may not be. Many people are still uninfected after several months, or even years. It seems that the risk of infection rises when the person becomes ill. Before then the risk may be much lower. You may want to be tested yourself. If you are positive, neither of you need to take as many precautions. If you are negative, then the following is sensible:

1. Use a thick strong condom carefully—see earlier in the chapter—with a spermicidal preparation containing nonoxynol.[28] This has two functions. First, the spermicide may damage some virus particles. Secondly, the extra lubrication can reduce the risk of a tear, and natural lubrication may be a bit lacking for a while if you are both on edge at first.

2. You may want to reduce the frequency of your lovemaking, but be sensible. Stopping altogether may cause terrible tensions and actually result in a rushed mistake. Arousal may

be much stronger after abstinence and then it is not as easy to be careful. Do not make love while a woman is menstruating, if she is positive, as the blood will probably contain virus.

3. Deep kissing, where saliva may pass from one mouth to another, is probably not a good idea. Dry kissing carries a much, much lower risk. Oral sex is not sensible.

4. An infected woman should probably avoid pregnancy as there is a significant chance that any child born may also be infected.[29] So use a second method of contraception as well, e.g. the pill, or consider sterilisation very seriously.

We have looked at the whole issue of the spread of AIDS and ways to reduce the risks of getting infected, but we have never been faced with a disease which confronts us with so many conflicting moral choices to do with rights and freedom. Some of these issues threaten to tear society apart. We consider the most important of these in the next chapter.

7

Moral Dilemmas

The reason why AIDS is such a sensitive issue is because it touches on so many different aspects of conscience and morality: sexuality and sexual behaviour, freedom of the individual versus protection of society, care for others, euthanasia, treatment or testing by force, suicide, and use and abuse of drugs, to name only a few.

Euthanasia—a word to those who care for others

Yesterday I went to see a man dying at home. He asked me to kill him as an act of mercy. Euthanasia literally means 'mercy death'. In some countries it is legal, but in the United Kingdom it is illegal. Why did he ask? He is in no pain because of the proper use of painkillers, nor is he feeling sick. He has a very slight cough but is eating quite well. His mind is superbly clear but he is confined to bed and unable to walk. He knows he is dying and talks about it freely without fear. He has a faith and feels he knows where he is going.

He feels his life has lost its meaning. He feels he would rather be dead than continue like this. Some doctors in some countries would have killed him, and a third of family doctors in the United Kingdom might have, but for the law.[1] He would have been in a coffin by this morning. But look at the situation more closely: many different emotions are tied up together and need separating. He feels a terrible burden on his wife. They have had a happy marriage and this is destroying it. He has always led the way and now feels helpless. It is rare for someone to ask for euthanasia without 'burden on other people' being a major factor. If we give way and agree, we are then killing people because they feel they are too much trouble to family or friends. This is a hazardous course. We are then killing people because—say—a friend, partner, or child is getting fed up and resentful. When do you agree that the patient is too much of a burden on others, or disagree and say that others are coping fine? Sometimes I am asked to 'put someone away' admit them into a hospital or a hospice. Tensions are rising at home or there is no love lost in a relationship—it has been non-existent for years. The carer takes me to one side: 'I want him put away somewhere.' My first priority is that if someone wants to die at home, that person should be able to do so.

Therefore it is vital to provide care and support for relatives and friends to enable that to happen. There are times when we have to admit someone to a hospital for 'social reasons' which usually means the collapse of support at home. You cannot force people to care, nor are they always physically able to. However, one tries if at all possible to create a situation where the sick person's wishes are observed. An atmosphere of resentment, hostility, or tension produces unimaginable, unbearable pressures for someone who is dying. They often feel compelled to agree to going back to a hospital or even to ask for euthanasia.

The second major reason why people make this request is because of depression. I am not talking about natural sadness. To feel overwhelmed by sadness because of leaving loved ones, losing strength, and because of dashed hopes for the future is normal. It is abnormal to be spectacularly cheerful in such circumstances. Natural sadness is not depression. Depression is where feelings of sadness are out of all proportion to the situation. This exaggeration of natural emotion can be caused by all kinds of things including hormonal changes or chemicals in the body, and needs urgent treatment. Occasionally it is because lots of minor or major sad events have been brushed under the carpet for years without tears or low spirits. Behind the mask of ecstatic happiness there has been a growing mountain of grief for losses of various kinds. Eventually something happens and the mask cracks. The person cannot hold back the flood any longer. An exam is failed or the car is written off and the person has a major breakdown. People think they are 'off balance,' crying all the time for no obvious reason because they fail to look deeper to the root of major hurts and losses over a long period of time. Many have breakdowns in adult life because of childhood sexual abuse by a parent, for example—a deadly secret that has never been shared.

When someone is depressed, he or she always loses a sense of self-worth. Everything is useless and hopeless. Everything is an effort and may result in self-centredness or a feeling of being a burden. Suicide is becoming common in the United Kingdom.[2] If a person is very ill, that person will be unable to commit suicide without help. Would you sit and watch a friend who was depressed, but not physically ill, swallow one hundred tablets without trying to stop him or her? No. Nor would you give the person a bottle of pills if he were unable to walk. You see, depression is quite common when you are unwell. When the body is physically low it can affect the brain so that you feel an exaggerated sadness. Sometimes this is due to chemical imbalances in the blood caused by the illness.

Someone who approves of euthanasia must be absolutely sure that the person is only naturally sad, and not depressed. Even psychiatrists find it hard to distinguish the two.[3] Depression always lifts given time, with or without treatment, although treatment may shorten its course.[4] Are you really going to kill someone who is emotionally ill, who may feel differently in a few weeks? Are you going to kill someone who is feeling a burden, when he may be under pressures you do not understand from others? Yes, you may say, because you feel his quality of life is awful, but who are you to judge? Many people find being with someone who is ill or disabled, emotionally traumatic and disturbing. Many panic phone calls come from people—even professional carers—who cannot cope with their own anxieties.[5] You may be in danger of killing someone because you have a problem coping and this colours your reaction to the person's request. With your own reaction, the patient's mood, and subtle pressures from others, you are on dangerous ground to do an irreversible, eternal act.

If you are still unconvinced, consider this if you are a doctor or a nurse—especially if you are regularly caring for people who are dying. A nurse visiting dying patients may get a reputation as an 'angel of death'. You know death is never far away when she visits someone in the next bed to you or a neighbour on your street.

Often people are too weak to swallow medicines shortly before they die and the last dose or two has to be given by injection.[6] Sometimes a nurse draws the curtains, injects someone near death, and five minutes later the person is dead. The drug is still largely sitting in the muscle where it was injected. Very little has reached the blood. The injection did not kill the person—he was just much, much closer to death than anyone realised. But it looks awful.

'That lovely doctor came into our house, took one look, and gave him an injection to put him out of his misery. He died two hours after. You wouldn't even let a dog suffer like that. It was the injection that put him to sleep.' Nothing will persuade the person otherwise. She is convinced euthanasia was committed.

Doctors and nurses are in a vulnerable position. If ever there was the faintest suspicion, grounded in fact, that foul play had been committed, we would lose all trust from patients and other colleagues. I cannot warn you more strongly. If you practise euthanasia as part of care of the dying you will cut your own throat, bring into disrepute yourself and the whole of terminal care, which scares many people anyway.

From my own perspective, to harm a patient is to break part of the ancient Hippocratic oath. As a doctor I understand how we are made. There is more to life than life. There is a mystery here. No one can create life, and life is to be respected. Abortion and other things have cheapened human life. I believe human life needs to be treated with the highest regard. I will never commit euthanasia and I believe the man I mentioned at the beginning of the chapter was actually relieved when I told him so. I took away an unbearable pressure.[7] It was not an option. If I had said that I was willing to do it, he would then have been faced with a ghastly sense of obligation. This man was unusual in any case. Most people who ask for euthanasia do so because of inadequate relief of pain and other symptoms. With proper control of symptoms and accurate information, the terrible fears about what will happen as they get worse melt away.[8]

Fortunately those attempting euthanasia often fail. Even doctors. I remember coming on a ward one day to see a patient, looking at the drug chart and being amazed to see that three vast overdoses of a particular drug had been given only hours apart to this person without her consent or knowledge. Not even a cry for euthanasia. Fortunately she survived and died peacefully in her own time a week or two later. The staff had been unable to cope with their own distress. Let's stop playing God in secret, behind closed doors, and start giving back to people control over their own lives, with dignity, self-respect, and respect for human life.

Withholding treatment

We need to make a careful distinction between withholding treatment and euthanasia. Making a carefully planned decision not to start a particular treatment, or to stop one that may be artificially prolonging life or directly causing distress in someone who is near death and for whom the possibility of recovery is extremely remote, is not euthanasia. Relatives, friends, the patient himself, and staff can be involved in the decision although responsibility for it must always rest firmiy with the treating doctor.

Examples include the decision of an AIDS patient not to continue with radiotherapy or chemotherapy for extensive Kaposi's sarcoma, or not to be mechanically ventilated.[9] An AIDS patient may decide that he cannot bear the thought of another long struggle with many tests and special treatments for his next pneumonia, and decides to stay at home to die.[10] Radical, mutilating surgery may be declined by a cancer patient. Most people with cancer or AIDS die of chest infections. Pneumonia used to be called the 'old man's friend' because it allowed a stricken body finally to die peacefully. It may not always be appropriate to leap in with aggressive treatments. It is not appropriate to give cardiac massage and mouth-to-mouth assistance to an eighty-four-year-old woman who is extremely ill from a wide variety of other illnesses if she has a heart attack and her heart stops. Most attempts to resuscitate such persons fail. Of those that are 'brought back to life' many die before ever leaving the hospital. With the elderly the success rate is even lower. What are we playing at? A terrible way to die. There is a time and place for resuscitation and for just letting someone go.

People who have problems with this are usually scared of death. Death is seen as failure. They may be too emotionally attached to allow the person to go. Failure to use common sense in this area, failure to see death as a natural conclusion to the process of living drives many doctors—especially surgeons—to absurd lengths, ridiculous operations, and ever more exotic procedures designed to fight to the end whatever the costs. It is the doctor who is treating his own problem. Doctors often feel guilty because they raised hopes too high in the first place, the person gets worse and is justifiably puzzled, upset, and angry. The doctor feels under pressure to do something. (See p. 158.)

The result is often catastrophic. Terminal care teams pick up the pieces every week of such inappropriate behaviour. We must learn to allow the body to die. Every year new medical methods make death more elusive. We can now keep someone's body warm and healthy for many years without any brain. This is not medicine. This is unhuman science gone mad.

Suicide

Suicide is a common terminal event in people with AIDS—usually early in the illness[11]—but also tragically in people who have had a positive test result, especially if counselling afterwards was poor. This is why the new over-the-counter home testing kits which will be available soon are so dangerous. They have just been outlawed in the United Kingdom. A small but growing number are also committing suicide because they fear they have AIDS.[12] The other day a patient on an AIDS ward went home suddenly for the weekend and gassed himself using the exhaust of his car and a piece of tubing. When someone has lost his job, been thrown out of his home, been rejected by family and deserted by friends, it is not surprising he feels suicidal. Glances in the street and people muttering in the shops are easily imagined but may be quite real. News of AIDS spreads only too fast. We need to show that we really care and go out of our way to make infected people feel accepted, loved, and welcome. If someone is depressed it may be wise to ask him if he has ever thought of harming himself. You may be afraid of putting a wrong idea into the patient's head. You won't, but the answer is vitally important.

If the person says no, then suicide is much less likely. If the person says yes, then ask if they have thought out how they would do it. Most people have not. Someone who can describe to you with clinical detachment and in great detail exactly how he would kill himself is probably at great risk.

His doctor should be told, and he should be persuaded to seek medical help. Tablets and other parts of his plan should be destroyed. Often a suicidal patient has secret supplies. Threats of suicide can be a most powerful means of blackmail, however: 'If you leave me I shall throw myself under a train,' or 'If you go on holiday for weeks I shall probably drown myself. I won't be here when you get back.'

But like euthanasia, suicide is harder than people think, and the after-effects of an attempt can be horrible.

Suicide is often attempted as a cry for help. Particularly tragic is the person who takes twenty paracetamol tablets expecting to go off to sleep. After most of a day has passed, the person walks into casualty looking sheepish. The psychiatrist is asked to help. It was a cry, not a serious attempt, but the liver is now permanently damaged. Within a few days the person begins to die an awful death and is dead in a week. Many over-the-counter preparations contain paracetemol.[13]

AIDS testing without consent or mandatory testing

At the time of writing, a doctor in England who tests someone's blood without prior agreement could be struck off the medical register or prosecuted. However at a recent meeting of the British Medical Association most doctors present voted to do so under special circumstances—usually where they believe the patient's life may be at risk through not knowing that he or she has AIDS.[14]

The reason for these rules is to protect people who are infected. People with the infection need protection because although they may be free of any signs of illness for years, it is a hard secret to keep and the knowledge that you are positive can be totally devastating. People lose jobs, houses, friends, and partners as a result. They cannot get a mortgage, a car loan, or life insurance.[15] Life insurance companies are worried. American actuaries have reckoned that AIDS claims could cost United States companies $50 billion by the year 2000.

The other reason for the regulations is strangely the ultimate protection of society. Control of sexually-transmitted diseases has always been hard because people are reluctant to seek help so the disease is untreated and more people are infected. They are afraid of being judged by doctors and nurses. The whole ethos of a clinic is to go overboard in providing a non-judgemental, tolerant, relaxed, attractive atmosphere with easy access and long opening hours. The aim is to entice people who may be infected so they can be tested, and infections cured. A clinic in West London prides itself in being busy with people coming from large distances because of its nice atmosphere. Judgemental, condescending behaviour puts people off and they continue to infect other people. It drives the problem underground, endangering the health of a whole community. And all this was before AIDS.

If people were afraid that while attending a hospital clinic for an unrelated reason or while in a hospital being prepared for an operation, a sample of blood would routinely be tested for HIV, there would be one result: they would be too scared to seek medical help at all. People would die at home of appendicitis or even from treatable chest infections as a result of developing AIDS. The entire problem would go underground.

In one respect, however, the problem of AIDS is unlike

syphilis. If you can make a diagnosis of syphilis you can treat it, cure it, and protect the whole community. With AIDS there is no cure and the person always remains a risk to sexual partners. Driving the problem underground will certainly deny infected people access to normal medical care but it will probably not spread the disease that much faster. If the person attends for his hernia operation and is not routinely tested, he will go away none the wiser. Spread is then stopped only when full-blown AIDS is diagnosed from a strange infection or tumour, the person is counselled, and then changes his behaviour.

While the arguments *against* testing without consent are very strong indeed, the situation is not clear cut and the opposite views are going to grow in strength.[16] Protecting those who are infected is praiseworthy, but it may put others at risk. For this reason there are various Acts of Parliament in England that allow a person to be detained against his will if, in the opinion of a doctor, he is likely to endanger the health of others.[17] In the United States, these matters are being debated, state by state. In Illinois, by the end of 1988, it was legal for any physician to test patients undergoing treatment for HIV and to disclose the result to sexual partners or others thought to be at risk. Colorado and Missouri are very likely to implement similar measures.

Take the plight of a surgeon: should he not know when to take special care not to cut or scratch himself? It would be wrong for him to refuse to operate on someone who was ill and needed surgery, but what about someone wanting cosmetic surgery or even a sex change operation?[18] Is it right for someone who may know he is positive to ask a surgeon to take that risk when the patient's own life is not at stake?[19] Most emergency rooms now use paper strips to close minor wounds instead of stitches. In most cases with small wounds the results are just as good, if not better, than with stitches because stitches can get infected and cause a body reaction. A stitch or two may reduce the risk of a slight scar, especially in a young girl, unless the cut is deep or the patient is particular. But if someone has the virus, is the risk of stitching acceptable? Metal surgical clips can be used to close wounds after surgery. It has been suggested that they should be used with all high risk patients.[20] Just how many people will need medical care for AIDS over the next twenty years? Millions. Maybe seventy-five million in Africa alone.[21] Even if the risk from an individual patient is small, the risk can multiply millions of times.

The fact is that a large number of doctors and nurses worldwide are going to die of AIDS over the next decade or two unless there is a cure or a vaccine. Accidents with needles and during operations happen in every hospital every day—most too minor to report but still capable of transmitting infection.[22] Years ago such people often died in the course of duty, from tuberculosis, for example. But today it is incredibly rare. A fireman occasionally dies fighting a fire or a policeman in trying to save a man from drowning. Doctors and nurses rarely die from their patient's infections. This will not be so in the future. Britain's Trades Union Congress (TUC) has suggested routinely screening everyone who is admitted to a hospital to protect health care workers[23] although at the moment the risks are much higher from private lifestyles of members of staff.[24]

The argument in favour of selective testing without consent is that the alternative is to assume that everyone is positive and take incredibly elaborate precautions. Time may be wasted and lives lost.

A certain man is known to have been a drug addict up to a year ago and needs open heart surgery. Treating him as 'presumed HIV infected' adds enormously to the operation cost. The theatre has to be closed for cleaning afterwards.[25] A twenty-minute operation took two and a half hours of theatre time recently when all the procedures were followed.[26]

A simple test could save all that nine times out of ten.

Some countries are now preparing to force certain groups of people to be tested. Military recruits in the United States of America army have all been tested routinely for some time. Iraq is testing all long-term visitors to the country. Bavaria in West Germany is testing groups as a matter of law. I think many people are going to disappear rather than be tested.

However, I am convinced that unless a cure is found quickly, HIV testing will become part of the routine work-up before any operation. I think it will be justified by surgeons as in the patient's interests on the grounds that fevers and chest infections after the operation may be mistaken for normal consequences of anaesthetic and surgery, correct treatment will not be given and the patient could suffer. At least one surgeon in the United Kingdom is regularly testing people for HIV regardless of whether they are in a risk group or not. This is without consent.

I also think HIV testing will be done on many patients in hospital wards with unusual symptoms of almost any kind. AIDS is such a complex disease because it opens the body up to so many other kinds of illnesses. It must therefore be on a physician's list of possibilities in an enormous number of people who are ill these days. Without the test the diagnosis will have to be made by excluding every other possibility, by which time the patient may be dead. This becomes vitally important as soon as we have any AIDS drugs that start to look as though they really might be effective. Once this happens, testing without consent will become widespread and justified on the grounds that prompt treatment could prolong or save life—although the real motive may be different.

It may seem shocking to test people for a disease without their knowledge but we have been doing it for years: blood testing for syphilis is common for similar reasons. It mimics such an enormous number of diseases. People are not always confronted with their result. In fact the vast majority of blood tests are done with what is called 'implied consent'. By agreeing to come into a hospital the person is accepting treatment. By agreeing to allow a blood sample to be taken 'for various things—like to see if you are anaemic' a person can often be tested for twenty or more different things. A diabetic woman develops severe thrush, a symptom of AIDS that can also be caused by badly controlled diabetes. The doctors think AIDS is highly unlikely and do not want to make her anxious by asking her permission to do a test and then leave her in suspense until the test result is back. So they may decide to test her anyway and only tell her the result if it is positive.

However, the great problem is keeping the result strictly

confidential. Medical teams must improve at this, especially family doctors, and occupational physicians in work places.[27]

Counselling following a positive test is vitally important. As we have seen, it is not uncommon for someone to kill himself following the discovery of a positive result.

So far we have looked only at testing of a person without consent in order to influence either the treatment given or the precautions taken. However, there is another moral dilemma: the testing of unmarked blood samples as part of an anonymous fact-finding exercise.

We have been in a crazy situation in the United Kingdom where we have not really had any idea at all how many people are infected. We knew only the majority of those who develop AIDS. Nor did we really know how the epidemic is spreading.

There is a way we will soon know. It is cheap and simple, breaks no confidence, and affects no individuals in any way at all. This way is to instruct various laboratories in certain hospitals not to throw their old blood bottles away—many keep them anyway for a week or so—but to remove all identifying markers on them and send them to the public health laboratory for AIDS testing. The result will be quick and helpful: maybe it will show that over a year the number of women infected at a London teaching hospital doubled whereas in East Anglia the number was constant. The only areas of the United Kingdom where such testing has occurred in any form has been at blood transfusion centres, where every unit given has been tested since 1985. This is helpful but we need more facts. Until now doctors and laboratories have refused to help on totally irrational grounds.[28]

They say it is immoral to test someone for AIDS and not tell them if the result is positive. Therefore no one should be tested unless the intention is to tell him the result. But this is a different situation where a group of people is being sampled anonymously. Anyone can ask for a test to be done at any time if he or she wants. No extra blood is taken and only existing blood samples are used so there is no discomfort or inconvenience. The United Kingdom government has now decided to carry out systematic, anonymous testing at regular intervals.[29]

The other problem area is mandatory testing, for example of engaged couples in Illinois. Mandatory testing is hard to enforce, whatever your opinion may be. In Illinois marriage applications in 1988 dropped by 67 per cent as couples went to other states to get married.[30]

Revenge sex and other situations

What do you do if someone you know is positive and has decided to get revenge on society by having sex with as many other people as possible? A man visiting New York woke up after a date to find 'Welcome to the AIDS club' written on his mirror. He is now infected.[31] A man was recently murdered in New York after announcing to the man he had just had sex with that he was positive. The murdered man had made the mistake of laughing.

Recently a newspaper reported a boy prostitute in London was taken out of circulation and into custody because he was determined to get others infected.[32] This report was hotly denied by social services.[33]

A drug addict in Norway 'infected fifty people after he discovered he had the disease.'[34] This opens up the broader issues of confidentiality: a businessman is positive and has no intention of telling his wife, who is wanting to have a baby. If she is positive, pregnancy could mean death for her and her child. Do you just sit back and wait for the inevitable? This whole area of law is confused: there are no test cases yet in the United Kingdom. The Public Health (Infectious Disease) Regulations of 1985 and the Act of 1984 could be interpreted as giving a hospital the authority via a magistrate to compulsorily detain such a person.

Human rights are always complex. You cannot have rights without responsibilities. You have a right to bring up your own children but you must not abuse that right by abusing your children. The businessman has a right to confidentiality but his wife has rights too. She has the right to live to seventy or more and not catch HIV. She has the right to be told and to choose about having a baby. Whose right is greatest? An expert on medical law, Professor Ian Kennedy, believes that doctors could be sued if they fail to inform an uninfected husband or wife even if forbidden to do so by the patient.[35] If someone is raped, should that person have the right to insist that the rapist is tested?[36]

I think many doctors are going to recognise that a small minority may be using their rights to confidentiality as a passport to injure and destroy others. If someone knows he or she is positive and sleeps with someone who is not, without warning them of the situation first, and that person becomes positive, it has been suggested that the man or woman concerned should be prosecuted for grievous bodily harm.[37]

The Solicitor General for Scotland, Mr Peter Frazer, has announced that people who maliciously or recklessly infect someone with the virus may be prosecuted for assault, under existing Scottish laws. A drug addict was jailed for three years for spitting in a policeman's eyes 'to give him AIDS'.[38]

A New York judge has ruled that damages can be claimed from a sexual partner if you can prove that he or she infected you and that the partner knew he or she was infectious and did not tell you. A lawsuit for a case of herpes involved a claim for over $1 million.[39] One man in Arizona faces two charges of assault and sodomy. This will change to a charge of murder if either victim dies.[40] In West Germany such an offender can be charged with manslaughter.[41]

Prosecution allows people infected as a result of crime to put in a claim to the criminal injuries compensation board. For the sake of the community, prostitutes should not be allowed to practise if they are positive. How many men do you think each prostitute services each year? According to a recent United Kingdom report, up to two hundred per week or ten thousand a year. A study of fifty London prostitutes showed that nine out of ten thought there should be compulsory testing, and eight out of ten thought that a prostitute should be prosecuted if she worked knowing she was infected.[42]

It has been suggested that all people who are infected should be issued identity cards. Such a proposal has been roundly condemned because of experiences of retaliation and discrimination in the community.[43]

It is incredibly worrying that a number of people who know they are positive have returned to clinics only a few weeks later with a new infection of gonorrhoea.[44] Some have got this from promiscuous behaviour without a condom. They are wilfully infecting others. These are questions that doctors and governments are going to be faced with sooner than they realise.[45]

Telling the truth?

Two months ago I went to visit someone who was dying at home. I was accosted in the hallway by an anxious relative who was convinced that the only reason I was there was to tell the patient his diagnosis and that he was dying. Nothing I could say would convince this relative otherwise. She was terrified. In fact we found as a team that working with this family became impossible. The sticking point was that I said that although I would never mention his probable death unless he himself asked, I was not prepared to lie to him. I might give an indirect answer such as, 'Why do you ask?' or, 'You don't seem to be getting any better, do you?' but I was not prepared to say, 'Of course not, don't be so stupid!'

The reason is very simple: trust. One day he would have realised I was lying. Actually, as far as I could see from what he said, he knew he was dying anyway—most people do. Most people with cancer or AIDS have guessed what is happening long before they are told. People aren't that stupid. Having established myself as a liar whenever it suits me to save embarrassment or calm fear, what happens when the person asks if they will die in terrible pain? This time I answer truthfully—but will I be believed? Often when people are first referred to us, they are convinced they are going to 'suffocate to death'. They may have terrible nightmares and be consumed with fears. Every time they get a cough we get a telephone call—the reason is overwhelming fear of what may be around the corner.

The truth is that no one suffocates to death these days. Hospices have advanced our care of those with lung disease enormously over the last twenty years. That is the truth—but will the public believe it? Fear of death can be worse than the dying itself.

Trust is the most powerful tool a doctor has. It is the reason why support teams and hospices are so successful. They inspire trust because they do not engage in the same frauds, cover-ups, and webs of petty deceit that are practised daily on the wards of every hospital. If only doctors realised that people see through it all!

The reason for dishonesty by doctors, and dishonesty by families and friends is simply this: we live in a society which likes to pretend that death does not exist. AIDS then hits us like a thunderbolt straight between the eyes, because it brings us face to face with death, and all our deepest fears. But before we take a look at the whole life/death issue, I want to turn to just one more moral dilemma which I get faced with every day as a church leader. The question people ask is this: Do I agree with those who say that AIDS is the wrath or judgement of God?

8

Wrath or Reaping?

Wrath of God?

Is AIDS the wrath of God? I am asked what I think about this issue almost every day, because I am a church leader as well as a doctor and often find myself talking to churches and other church leaders about AIDS. It is one of those areas where you know that any phrase or sentence you say or write could be turned into a banner headline of whatever kind the editor thinks will sell the most papers or media time. I am also aware that you may be one of the hundreds in bookshops who will judge this book by whether you agree with what I say. You will either buy it or want to burn it. Whatever I say there may be ten of the former and one hundred of the latter. You will either say I am judgemental or a heretic or a liberal. What follows is a personal view from a church leader who takes seriously what the Bible says.

In the mid-1980s medical advice filtering through the media was that AIDS was spread only by anal sex. Anal sex was defined as an unnatural act that caused bleeding and infection of the partner. The public impression was that unless you were gay you could not get AIDS. Clergymen and church leaders then grabbed their Bibles and began a series of private and public pronouncements in the United States and the United Kingdom denouncing homosexuality, listing plagues described in the Old and New Testaments, and declaring that this was obviously God's plague on homosexuals[1]—obviously as it only appeared to affect them.

This reaction has been fuelled by a distorted perception of sexual sin which is part of our culture and not part of Jesus' own sayings. Before you reject this out of hand, you who are churchgoers, read on. Incidentally, it is usually men who are so vehement in condemning the homosexual man. Women are far more tolerant. Yet the same men are more tolerant of two lesbians. Why? Does God find sex between two men more offensive than between two women or an adulterous relationship? AIDS is almost unknown in lesbians.

First, those church leaders are now acutely embarrassed. They are on record as declaring this is God's judgement on homosexuals although there are now known to be many more women and babies infected than there ever were homosexual men. They fire salvoes at the visible tip of the iceberg, ignoring the millions of women, children, and heterosexual men beneath the surface. The 'wrath' theology is then adjusted to include all who are promiscuous—again acutely mistaken.[2] What do you say to those millions of children who may die in Africa or elsewhere as a result of medical treatments (blood and injections)? Children are dying in the United Kingdom, in America, Romania, Soviet republics and many other countries.

Nothing new

'Wrath of God' theories are nothing new. Several centuries ago a plague for which there was no cure swept the known world. Signs of infection were absent sometimes for many years and controversies raged over which country it had all started in. It was spread by sexual intercourse. I am referring to syphilis which, as we have seen, only became curable with the advent of penicillin in 1944.

Church leaders at the time declared it was the wrath of God. This had two effects: search for a cure was inhibited or actively discouraged—after all you were interfering with the natural course of judgement. Also, those with syphilis were treated in a less sympathetic way: 'It is their own fault and they put society at risk.'

A friend of mine spent some months in a certain developing country in 1974. Many men came into the hospital clinic where he was working because they had difficulty passing water. Gonorrhoea infection had caused scarring and narrowing of the delicate tube (urethra) inside the penis. Sometimes these people would have full bladders and be in great discomfort. The way to treat this is by pushing a series of rods into the penis, each one larger than the one before, to dilate the stricture. This causes excruciating, unbearable pain unless you use local anaesthetic cream. It is so painful that most surgeons in the United Kingdom do this under a general anaesthetic. The cream was stacked on the shelves and men were screaming out in agony. Greatly shocked by this my friend asked why the pain-killing cream was not being used, or a full anaesthetic. The answer was that this was an immoral disease and the person must be punished. I wish it were not so but these people had been influenced by atmosphere and culture imported by church missionaries. What has that appalling attitude got in common with the way of Jesus?

You may recoil from this but you must realise that in the United States and the United Kingdom parts of the church are currently fostering the very same attitudes to the very same kind of epidemic. The words are not the same, but the same atmosphere of rejection of the person is there.

Be consistent

Be consistent: if AIDS is the wrath of God then syphilis was too. I cannot see any difference between AIDS and any other disease from the medical point of view. The agent of the wrath of God is often recorded as being an angel in the Old and New Testaments. It is portrayed as a supernatural intervention that is selective. Contrast this with AIDS, caused by a virus which has probably existed in some shape or form for thousands of years. It has existed in animals for a long time, and maybe also in humans. The explosive spread—as with syphilis—has been along the lines of international travel and sexual relationships. It behaves according to the rules of every other infection with its own particular preferences and effects.

As I said at the beginning of the book—what is so special about AIDS? Nothing. You have been misinformed. The only thing that makes it unusual is that you may not know you are infected for years and when people get full-blown AIDS they all eventually die. The reaction of extreme fear associated with AIDS is unusual. But fear, lack of signs, and high death rate from a viral disease are not the same thing as God's judgement. For me, the key to the whole thing is the attitude of Jesus.

Caught in the act

At the crack of dawn Jesus was at the temple teaching a huge crowd. Sitting and standing, leaning against the walls, they listened quietly as Jesus sat down. It was still cold under the stark sunlight and the vast stones were damp with dew. Jesus' voice quietly rose and fell. There was silence apart from an occasional cough or the bleat of an animal outside.

Suddenly all heads turned at the sound of a great commotion. Twenty or thirty people burst in shouting and screaming. Jesus stopped. He was used to such interruptions. They happened almost every day—either by friends bringing someone wanting to be healed or by the authorities hoping to provoke a confrontation and arrest him.

A woman was thrown down at his feet. She and Jesus stood up together. She had been discovered in bed half an hour ago with another woman's husband. Caught in the act. The men who brought her were furious, seething with anger. They demanded a response from Jesus: 'The law says we must drag her away, pick up rocks and boulders, and stone her to death. What do you say?'

It was yet another trap and Jesus knew it. If he had agreed with the law they would have dragged him away and stoned him for being judgemental and severe. If he had not agreed, they would have arrested him for being too liberal.

Who's perfect?

Jesus did nothing at all. He said nothing at all. The mob were pressing in, repeating their question over and over again, pushing and shoving aggressively. All the while the people in the court were watching and waiting. Tension was rising. Someone was going to get hurt—either Jesus or the woman was likely to be lynched. The very forces who could have prevented it were standing right there in the temple.

Jesus knelt down on the ground under the harsh glare and threats of the men and was silent. He wrote on the ground with his finger. The shouting and abuse got louder.

Jesus stood up and looked at them. Instantly there was quiet. Jesus looked into the eyes of each man standing there. 'You who are so perfect, you who have never cheated anyone, lied, or been selfish, you who are always so perfectly loving and kind, you who never lose your temper, you who are so generous, you who have never had a lustful thought ... Yes, you come forward now, come and take a stone, come and throw it at this woman. Be the first to throw.'[3]

Jesus looked at each man in turn, but they shrank away, uncomfortable under his gaze. He knelt down again and stared at the ground as he wrote with his finger in the dust. The older men began to peel off from the crowd and disappeared down the temple steps. One at a time they left in silence. Gone were the shouts, the threats, and the abuse. Eventually none was left—only those who had come to hear Jesus teach.

No condemnation

Jesus stood up. The woman was still standing there, her head hung in shame, humiliation, and embarrassment. She stood afraid, unable to move, afraid of the men waiting outside, afraid of what Jesus was thinking.

Jesus looked at her. Spies in the crowd were about to slip out and report that Jesus had been trapped: he had given himself away as a liberal by letting an adulterer off free.

Jesus said to the woman, 'Where are they? Has no one condemned you?'

'No one, sir?' she replied. Jesus then said two vitally important things: 'Then neither do I condemn you?' and then he added: 'Do not sin again.'[4]

Men had caught a man and a woman making love. One of them was married to someone else. They let off the man and judged the woman. Double standards: their own they excused, the other they condemned. As far as they were concerned, they were just expressing the natural wrath and displeasure of God, but Jesus rejected their whole attitude. Jesus was concerned not just with actions but also with attitude. As far as he was concerned, to have an adulterous fantasy could be as bad as committing adultery.[5] One person may be no worse than the other—just one had the opportunity and the guts to actually do it, the other no opportunity or was too afraid.

The man who is angry with his brother could be as bad as someone who kills. Read what Jesus said for yourself.[6] Actions are not everything. What goes on in the secret places of your heart and imagination is also vitally important.[7]

Never do it again

Jesus did not distinguish between the subtleties of wrong. We are all wrong. We have all done wrong or thought wrong. None of us is perfect.[8] As the only perfect man, he was the only person who had the perfect right to condemn the woman, but he did not. Why not?

Because he loved her and understood himself what it was like to be tempted.[9]

Did he excuse her? Not at all. Did he encourage her? Not at all. Did he allow her to get off free? Not at all. He rebuked her. He told her she had been wrong. He told her never to do it again. He told her never to do anything else wrong again. 'Go and learn from your lesson' was his message.

They were *all* wrong: the men were hypocrites. When Jesus said that, every single one realised it was true. Every single one of them had had lustful thoughts and fantasies about other people's wives at some time or other. Every single one of them, if they were really honest, knew that deep down inside they were not as nice as they tried to appear on the outside. Only they and their families knew what they were really like at home with the door closed. Only they knew how selfish and mean they could be sometimes. Their own consciences convicted them, and they backed away. In some ways they were no better and no worse than the woman. If she deserved stoning, so did they.

The trouble is that in every town, in every village, in every church, in every country—and maybe in your home, maybe in yourself—there are attitudes just as revolting to Jesus as the attitudes of that crowd: judgemental, harsh, intolerant, vicious, cruel, and bitter. No! you may say. I'm not like that, nor is anyone I know. Consider this then:

Banner headlines

What is your attitude to a clergyman who is prosecuted for sexually abusing children?

Banner headlines hit the United Kingdom recently over several vicars and a church worker who were charged with sexually assaulting children. National Childwatch—featured in September 1987 on the BBC documentary *Diane's Children*—has dossiers on other clergy they are hoping to bring to the courts. The children involved were all boys in the churches concerned, whether members of youth clubs, choirboys, or whatever.[10]

Diane Core, who runs National Childwatch,[11] was so appalled by all this that she wrote to the Archbishop of Canterbury to request a meeting. National Childwatch feels that up until now the problem has been covered up or denied, although it may be affecting many churches. The point I am making here is: What is your attitude?

So much for vicars assaulting small boys. What is your attitude to a married priest who is discovered in bed with a parishioner's wife, or in a public toilet with his trousers and pants down, having anal intercourse with another man?

In most circles inside and outside the church, the reaction to all these things is shock and outrage. You say it is despicable because of his position. That person has undoubtedly lost his ability to lead a congregation. He has been living a charade, a façade behind which lies a guilt-ridden twilight world or else he has rewritten the rule book to make his conduct compatible with his faith. But in your sweeping anger you have condemned him. Your outrage is identical to that angry crowd confronting the woman.

Double standards

Clergy do not have some super gift of God that keeps them perfect. In fact the Bible does not distinguish between clergy and laity at this point. We are all a royal priesthood.[12] All who claim to be Christians are called to live up to our calling.[13] None of us is exempt. There are no double standards. As you would expect, there are minimum standards for life and conduct laid down for those appointed to positions of leadership in the church and certainly such responsibility brings special accountability. However these minimum standards such as managing his household well, being sober and self-controlled, are no more or less than those expected of all of us. It is interesting that the lists of qualifications are all to do with character, not gift or experience.[14]

Individuals who behave in the ways listed above need to be accepted as people, while we may not necessarily accept everything they do or say. As people we find this almost impossible—we either accept the person and what he or she does, or land up rejecting the behaviour and the person. It is not what you say, but the way you say it that can be most important. Some people say they care about drug addicts but give out an atmosphere of coldness. Some people say that as Jesus loved all people, they too accept all people, but still display deep-rooted prejudices at every turn. You who are perfect—you cast the first stone.

God calls us to accept all people and to extend his love to them regardless of whether or not we agree with what they do. Impossible you say. How can this be reconciled with God's absolute standards? Jesus came for all men. Not for the perfect but to invite 'sinners to repentance'.[15] Did Jesus come to bring forgiveness and peace to the repentant murderer? Of course he did. God's love and mercy is so unbelievably great that if even Hitler had genuinely repented and given his life to God in that bunker in 1945, the Bible tells us he would be in heaven now. Death-bed conversion is real. The thief crucified next to Jesus was told that within a few hours he would be with Jesus 'in paradise'[16]

Judgement without tears is obscene

You may reject all this, you may go through the Bible quoting texts about God's wrath and anger. It is possible to be correct but horribly wrong. It is possible to be correct about God's displeasure but lack love. A well-known Christian leader once said that 'to speak of judgement without tears is obscene'. Where are your tears? Go and find your tears of grief for those who are suffering, dying and, you say, in line for judgement. When you have found your tears, then talk to me of judgement—but start with yourself.

Reaping natural consequences?

It is a fact of life that everything has consequences. If you drink and drive you may injure or kill yourself and others. If you sniff cocaine you may get a hole inside your nose—the nose was not designed for cocaine. If you line your lungs with tobacco tar you can get a chronic irritation which may result in coughs and cancer. If you eat badly-cooked chicken you can get food poisoning. If you sleep with someone who is not a virgin, you could catch a number of illnesses which he or she may have got from a previous partner.

These things are so obvious. Cause and effect is also a central theme in the teaching of Jesus. The Bible teaches that we are creatures of choice. We are not automatons. We are free to choose God's way or our way. If that were not so there would be no point in telling us how to live because we would be unable to respond in any other way at all. But with freedom comes responsibility. The Bible teaches that each of us will have to give account one day for everything we have said, thought, done, should have done, and did not do.

The Christian position is that within the Bible our loving Father has recorded guidelines for healthy, stress-free, fulfilled living: 'How to be healthy and whole.' So what is the Christian view of sex? Here is a personal view.

Unlimited sex

Sex was invented to be enjoyed. It is one of the most amazing experiences God gave mankind. In God's plan, he intended a man and a woman to marry and in the context of that promise of commitment, care, love, and understanding, to explore together the kaleidoscope of physical love. God intended husband and wife to have unlimited sex: as often as they both would like and enjoy. Out of that beautiful loving relationship were to come children who would grow up feeling loved and secure, with a mum and a dad, grandparents, aunts, uncles, and cousins. God loves families. He created human beings to belong to each other, and those whose families had died or were far away to be cared for if they wanted by other families or communities.

Our bodies were not designed for multiple sexual encounters. Such a lifestyle has consequences. It is physically unhealthy. Before AIDS, promiscuity was already becoming more and more unhealthy. It was fairly risky until the advent of antibiotics dealt with gonorrhoea and syphilis. Then some penicillin-resistant strains of gonorrhoea emerged, along with various other infections such as herpes and chlamydia (Pelvic Inflammatory Disease). Now we know that early sex and multiple partners can also cause cervical cancer. This was all before AIDS. Promiscuity has always been unhealthy. Now it can be fatal.

Emotionally, sleeping around has always been hazardous. The result is usually destabilisation of any semi-permanent or permanent relationship. Although polygamy was practised in the Old Testament, the track record of its success and happiness is disastrous. Read the story of Abraham.[17] Adultery usually has catastrophic consequences for one person at least. I have yet to meet anyone where it did not. Divorce, too, is nearly always a traumatic disaster leaving lifelong scars. Sleeping around fractures relationships and will always be emotionally risky, unless there are no relationships. If there are no relationships then nothing is at risk. A prostitute has no emotional investment in her client—nor her client with her—so there is no loss or trauma. However, there may develop a more sinister and deeper damage to the ability to form lasting loyal commitments. The risk is a lonely bankruptcy of friendship and support after middle life has sapped physical drives and taken its toll on attractiveness and vitality.

Sleeping with multiple partners can have permanent spiritual effects too. The Bible teaches clearly that sex is a wonderful experience and one of the deepest mysteries known to human beings. When a man and a woman sleep together, the Bible says they become 'one flesh'.[18]

Something has taken place which can never be undone. Sex was designed as the ultimate expression of exclusive covenant love between a man and a woman. Devoid of relationship it is robbed of its quality and enjoyment and becomes a mere mechanical sensation. No wonder many unmarried people reject sleeping around and choose celibacy. They see through the glamorous veneer to the emptiness beneath. Those who are promiscuous are often driven into further and further searches for the ultimate in sexual satisfaction. Once you have divorced the physical act from the whole-person experience you have no hope at all of true fulfilment. Women usually realise this more than men. None of these things will satisfy your heart. You have been cruelly deceived and there may be consequences.

The Christian position is that when we break any of God's designs for living we create tension in our relationship with him. God is perfect and cannot tolerate sin. Nor can he reward us with the warmth of his love and approval when we have turned our backs on his best for us. Sin affects your nearness to God if you are a Christian and prevents your finding God if you are not. There is nothing especially wrong in sexual sin although its effects can be very destructive of relationships and communities. As we have seen, there is one sense in which it is no more displeasing to God than any other sins against others. I feel I must say again that often we fall into absurd double standards. People reject homosexual acts or adultery as more wrong in some way than lying or cheating or stealing or being cruel or hating someone. There is no such distinction in the Bible when it comes to separation from God.[19] Sin is sin, the other differences are merely cultural values and must be rejected. The Bible teaches that we are all imperfect. We all think wrong, feel wrong, and do wrong. We all fall far short of God's standards. None of us deserves any reward or favours from God, and there is nothing we can do to earn his pleasure. That is why no one can turn and point the finger at someone with AIDS.

Impossible barrier

You can never be good enough. Human imperfections always remain an impossible barrier between us and God. Without Jesus Christ, you can no more put human beings and God together than olive oil and water: they always separate.

That is why Jesus said, 'I am the way and the truth and the life. No one comes to the Father except through me.'[20] There are, we are told, hundreds of ways to God. Maybe, but none of them leads you to a personal relationship with a God who is almighty, omnipotent, unknowable, unreachable, and untouchable. Other religions may promise some kind of ethereal consciousness, but that is no substitute for a personal relationship. The reason is obvious. Other religions say that closely following a certain formula for holiness will deal with your imperfection. If only it could. The best formulas in the world and the most ardent efforts might possibly get you a mile or two nearer God. The trouble is that our imperfections distance us from God by several light years! But even after a lifetime of devoted holiness, you would have a chasm of several million miles to cross.[21]

No wonder Jesus himself said he was the only way to oneness with God the Father. Christians believe the good news that God himself provided a rescue plan for mankind because significant movement by us in his direction was impossible. So God himself moved toward us and entered our time-space world. He came in human form as Jesus.

When Jesus died, that whole issue of separation was dealt with for all time. Every single thing that separated us—all the consequences of our wrong doing and wrong attitudes—were lumped on Jesus' shoulders. As a sacrifice for all time he, the perfect God-man, allowed himself to die for us so that we might be forgiven and released from the consequences of what we have done. The result is now a doorway—a narrow one—to union with God our Father. You enter the door not by justifying to God what a wonderful person you are, but by believing and accepting all Jesus came to do—and by making a decision to give your life to him in obedience.

Unless you really understand the way the Bible portrays this separation and how Jesus overcame it, you will never grasp what Jesus said to the woman and the accusing crowd that morning: they were all finished. None of them had the remotest hope of peace with God. The men and women in the crowd, the adulteress herself, they were all hopelessly blocked from a relationship with their Father. That is, outside of following, believing, and trusting in Jesus, the only way, the truth about God, and the means of finding the life of God.

Changed lives

To all those who accept Jesus as Lord and turn away from everything wrong (repent means to turn around), he has given a brand new life.[22] That is why Jesus told a would-be follower that he had to be 'born again.'[23]

When I became a Christian, in one sense I died.[24] Baptism is a symbol of my burial. When I rose out of the water it was a symbol of my new birth.[25] The Bible says I am now a new creation: 'The life I now have is not my life, but the life which Christ lives in me.'[26] This is another mystery.

When someone becomes a Christian, the results are often dramatic.

Parents or children become easier to live with. Marriages begin a new start. Friendships are transformed. A friend of mine who became a Christian invited all his friends to his baptism (we use a local swimming pool). They all turned up with their heavy metal leather jackets and boots. Two were so amazed at what had happened to their friend that when they saw it wasn't just a passing fad, they became Christians as well.[27] When you've seen the real thing, who wants a substitute? Ordinary people changed by something outside themselves.

A friend from the United States was saying last week that he became a Christian partly through his mother's conversion. She was dying of severe kidney disease. The poisons were steadily accumulating in her body. She was not a believer but went to a healing meeting. She was prayed for healing and felt she had been instantly healed. She went back to the clinic as usual. The doctors were amazed. All the results of medical tests on her kidneys had returned to normal. Life was never the same for her. She became a Christian, and so did her son some time later.

I met someone recently after an AIDS talk. He told me he had been a heroin addict until three or four years ago when he became a Christian. He broke the habit immediately and is now a leader in his church. This is not unusual. Jesus gives people power by the Holy Spirit when they become Christians.[28]

You can be free to choose God's way even though chained to all kinds of things—addiction, childhood memories, or parts of your own human nature. Jesus came to set you free. You choose to follow him and he does the rest. You exercise your will and he will give you all the resources you need.[29]

Father's love

After a meeting at a London medical school, I overheard a conversation between a medical student and a member of the hospital Christian union. She was basically asking herself why she couldn't believe in God. 'I admire you people. I wish I could believe. You have it all together. You know where you are going. It's all right for you.'

I joined in. I asked her if she really wanted an answer to that question because I believed God wanted to answer it for her. I told her that God loved her whether she believed it or not. I told her the story of Jesus and the woman at the well.[30] Jesus broke the taboos by asking her for a drink. He then told her to go and fetch her husband. She replied that she didn't have one. Jesus agreed with her: 'You have been married five times and the man you are now living with is not your husband.' She was shocked. How did he know? She rushed to the village to tell them about this man who knew everything about her.

Such insights can be a part of Christian life today. I prayed for a moment and then said that I felt that part of the reason this girl could not believe was because of her family. She had never known what it was to feel loved, especially by her father, and so could not accept that God could care about her, especially love her as a father.

She sat down and started to cry. Tears poured down her face as she started to talk about her childhood, not a particularly unhappy one, but one devoid of open affection. She was hurting, bruised, and wounded. I asked if she wanted me to pray for her emotions and her past. She did. Even before I prayed her eyes seemed to open and she found she believed deep down. But it is hard to trust a heavenly Father's love if you have never experienced an earthly father's love. After we had prayed she made it clear she wanted to give her whole life to God. She realised she had been living life her way and now wanted to live life God's way. She wanted to turn her back on the past and begin again. She gave her life to God in a very moving prayer. There were tears in my eyes and in her friend's when we had finished.

About a year later I found myself sitting next to her at a conference. Friends had told me previously how much she had changed, how much happier and fulfilled she was, and how her student friends had all been along to various things with her to try and puzzle it out.

Father's discipline

People who have never known love find it hard to accept love—whether from a friend, a spouse, or from God. Likewise, people who have never known the balanced firmness and discipline of a loving father and mother can never really understand the discipline, firmness, and standards of God.

Jesus loves all people, but not necessarily what people do. He got angry and violent with traders using the temple area to make money out of pilgrims. He walked through the stalls, tipping up the trestle tables and throwing their goods on the ground.[31] There was chaos: their best wares and coins were flying everywhere. Then Jesus came at them again, this time with a whip of cords to drive them right out of the temple.[32] 'Gentle Jesus meek and mild' is not the whole Jesus of the Bible. And yet he loved them.

Many of Jesus' words to religious leaders were aggressive and cutting with biting sarcasm and savage wit. Wherever he went he slaughtered hypocrisy, double standards, false religion, and disregard for God's holiness. Today we shrink from preaching on many of the things Jesus said because they are so strong.

The thing on which Jesus was strongest of all was love. 'Love your neighbour' is hard enough—particularly when the story of the good Samaritan shows us that your neighbour is whoever you come into contact with regardless of nationality, background, circumstances, or personal risk.[33]

Loving your neighbour is not enough

Jesus then made one of the most devastating commands that has ever been made. Loving our neighbour is totally inadequate. We are also called to love our enemies, to express God's perfect love to those who hate us, despise us, want to hurt us, and beat us up.[34] Jesus calls us to love those who rape us, cheat us, and those who twist and distort things we say. He commands us to pray for people who persecute us or spitefully use us. This is not a command to mere forgiveness—though that itself is painfully costly and hard at times. This is a command to actively, positively seek to express warmth, compassion, kindness, and understanding to those we humanly would hate and regard as our worst enemies. We are told to pray for their happiness. This was not idle talk: Jesus lived out his message all the way to his crucifixion.

This may seem objectionable, impossible, and bizarre—but it is what Jesus said. After all, even the most horrible people tend to be nice to their friends. What is so special about being nice to your friends? What is so remarkable about loving those who love you? Nothing at all. We are called to be a visual aid, an active demonstration, a living temple of God's supreme love. Even more amazing is that God's love for us is incalculably greater than our love for others—because God is infinite and perfect.

Just as we are commanded to love, regardless of response, in a way which is totally without conditions or strings attached, so God our Father loves all people regardless of their response to him.

Now you can see that God does not hate or reject people

because he does not like what they do. He weeps over our slowness, our obstinacy, our self-centredness, our stupidity.

When it all goes wrong

When God made creation, he designed man and woman to be physically united in a marriage covenant, to be perfectly loving and perfectly faithful. What happens when it all goes wrong? When people make each other's lives hell in a desperately unhappy marriage, when people cheat each other in adultery, when people sleep around without the covenant commitment of marriage, when people express their sexuality by torturing their partners for pleasure, when children are sexually seduced by adults.... When it all goes wrong, what is the response of our Maker?

Sadness and dismay is his response. Where others are being hurt or emotionally damaged the response is anger. Where people choose to ignore a relationship with him, the result is no relationship with him. A living death, a living hell. An eternal disaster of constant separation. It is not that God's will is for any to be separated from him,[35] but that God is holy. Outside Christ—which is our choice—there can be no reconciliation.[36]

So does God condemn the adulterer? Not at all. He is sad at separation from the one he loves that may result. Does God condemn the practising homosexual? Not at all. He is sad at the distance the sin creates. Does God condemn the hypocrite, the liar, or the person who is mean with money? No, he is sad that the person has missed the way. Does God condemn the person whose rages spill over into violence? No, he is sad that the person is driven by these things.

However, the Bible teaches us that God's sadness and God's anger are closely linked. God is furious at some of the things we do. God's anger is the result of his perfect holiness and justice expressed through creation. God, although our loving heavenly Father, can never compromise. Anger and judgement are the discipline sides of love, to those who refuse to turn away from what is wrong, and refuse to follow him.[37]

At the end of the day the tension between God's love and God's anger is difficult to understand. God is himself a mystery to the human brain limited in time and space to a four-dimensional world.

You reap what you sow.[38] If you sow a certain way of life, you will reap the consequences of it. This is not God's wrath or judgement. This is a normal part of living. God is a loving Father whose wish it is to see the whole of creation united with him again as was the original plan.[39]

It is not his desire to see anyone perish, but for all to come into their full inheritance:[40] life outside the limitations of space and time, a wonderful life forever free from anguish, pain, and suffering.

However, we are created in freedom, and with that come guidelines and responsibilities. With choices come consequences—some of which are, we are told, unpleasant. We are warned that we cannot always undo what we have done and the biggest consequence of all is having to face our Maker after death with our track record.[41] That may not be such a pleasant experience. It may be a terrible shock to those who thought God didn't even exist. But at that time there will be no further opportunities to undo what has been done. The result will be separation from God with all the time-space world stripped away. A continuation of a relationship—or a lack of it. There are people right now who are separated from God and know it. They need to be reconciled to him and experience the warmth of his love.

People think finding God as a father is very complicated. It is as simple as apologising to God in your own words for living life your way and agreeing to live life his way, turning your back on the past, acknowledging Jesus as Lord to be worshipped and obeyed, and trusting him for everything. That is the way to experience the love of God as your father. That is the way to find forgiveness and cleansing for all you have ever done wrong, and that is the way to receive the help, comfort, and power of the Holy Spirit.

There are others who are separated who have no idea at all. So consumed are they with earning money, building a business, or making a nice home that they pay no attention to the empty spaces inside. Many of these people finally start being real about themselves when confronted by their own imminent death.

If only I had known what I know now

People who become Christians in later life often say, 'If only I had known what I know now. I would not have got divorced. I would still know my kids. I wasted so much of my life. Why didn't anyone tell me before?' They prohably did, it just took a sudden jolt to shake them out of their complacency. Death of a friend, adultery by a wife or husband, death of a child, diagnosis of AIDS. With AIDS there is an added dimension. Maybe if the person had become a believer a decade ago, he would not be infected. He could still be alive in twenty years' time.

Quite often people simply have not heard before. We live in a post-Christian era with various outward trappings of Christian life left, often devoid of content. In the church we tend to think everyone knows what Christianity is—but in fact very few do. Saying a prayer or two when in trouble and going to church does not make you a Christian. Being a follower of Jesus is what makes you a Christian. Jesus said that even the devil believes. It is the desire above all else to do God's will that makes the difference. 'Whoever cares for his own safety is lost; but if a man will let himself be lost for my sake, that man is safe.'[42] In businesses we often talk of the cost benefit analysis. Is a project likely to be worthwhile? In the church we major on benefits, but when did you last hear a sermon about the cost? Jesus majored on the cost, just as he majored on choice, responsibility, accountability, and consequences.

Strong stuff

It was Jesus himself who said that if my right eye caused me to go wrong then I should pluck it out (figuratively speaking) and throw it away rather than 'be thrown into hell where the devouring worm never dies and the fire is not quenched.'[43] Strong words from the strongest man the world has ever seen. You may not like them and I may not like talking about this whole area, but it is part of the truth. To say otherwise is to make God out to be some amoral, ethereal substance, neither able to feel nor think. Some indescribable unknowable something-or-other as vague as energy or cosmos. My God is more than that: Author, Originator, Prime Mover, who created a conscious, moral, decision-making, spiritually aware creature capable of relationships. Man was made in God's own image, a creature to have a relationship with his Maker, who is revealed to him in terms of an ultimate relationship, that of Father to son or daughter.[44]

How do we respond?

So how do we respond in a practical way? Even those who passionately defend their promiscuity or homosexual sex on moral grounds concede that if I found a friend of mine, a leader of a church, was having an affair with another man's wife, I should tell him to stop. In fact I usually find people outside the church are even fiercer in speaking out against such behaviour than many in the church. Those in the church are expected to behave! If I ask why, they say that a clergyman must act in a moral fashion. I agree. The Bible is quite clear that those who call themselves Christians are called to be loving, kind, generous, honest, and either faithful to their spouses or celibate.[45] To remain single is shown to be a positive releasing decision because it frees the person enormously to be mobile, able to go wherever God wants.[46] The Bible is exceptionally clear in outlawing sex between unmarried people and sex between other people's spouses. Sex between two men or two women is considered in just the same way as sex between unmarried people. For those in the church it is forbidden. Sex between a son and his mother or a father and his daughter or with animals is also outlawed. In fact any form of sexual intercourse outside of marriage is utterly forbidden.[47]

Sex is not unique in this regard. To bear a grudge is also forbidden.[48]

To be moody and feel sorry for myself all the time is forbidden. To get drunk is forbidden.[49] The way of Jesus is the way of perfect love.[50]

This feels very negative—boundaries always feel negative. If

I tell my four-year-old son he can cycle around the park but must keep within sight of me, he will feel I am negative. Boundaries are essential. Any child psychologist will tell you what happens when children don't know their boundaries. They are always testing to find the limits of what is acceptable. When there are no limits—or worse, the limits always vary—the child becomes insecure and can grow up immature. He may also be constantly at risk through lack of supervision.

Boundaries for healthy living

Out-of-bounds areas are marked for our protection and safety. The Falklands war has left hundreds of square miles of deserted land surrounded by barbed-wire. The reason is that hundreds of thousands of tiny plastic explosive charges lie inches beneath the soil. Treading on one can cost you a leg or a foot. They cannot be detected because they contain no metal and they cannot be destroyed. Those areas will remain out-of-bounds for decades. It would be strange if there were no fences, no barbed-wire, no warning signs. You can climb over if you like. No one will stop you although they may shout at you not to be so stupid. You have been warned by people who care and by people who knew that your instinct would be to run over the beautiful inviting fields and meadows.

The out-of-bounds areas laid down for us are not some great negative moralistic statement, but warning signs: 'Enter here at your peril, it could cost you.' It will cost you. It may cost you emotionally, physically, psychologically, and will certainly cost you spiritually. When we flout what God has given us as guidelines for life, whether by being selfish, dishonest, gossiping, being unkind, or by being unfaithful or uncontrolled in our sexual lives, there are spiritual consequences. It creates tension in our walk or communion with him. It creates a barrier that can only be removed by confessing to God that we have been wrong and have disobeyed. This is the only route to forgiveness, cleansing, wholeness, and inner healing.[51]

In conclusion

In conclusion, then, my own view is that AIDS is not an expression of the wrath or judgement of God, but is a part of the world of cause and effect in which we live. When it comes to the practicalities of healthy living, the Bible confirms what common sense tells us: that we are not designed for multiple sexual encounters and there is another way to live. However, all with AIDS need unconditional care.

So having considered some of the questions about sexuality and moral codes, what about the other big issue of death? It's an issue I face as a terminal care doctor every week of my life. Death and dying are no strangers to me in cancer work, yet walking onto an AIDS ward for the first time was quite a shock. Unlike a cancer ward where at least a few are expected to be cured, here was a row of faces, of people, of lives, every one of whom was doomed. Not a hope of cure in their lifetimes, bar a strange miracle or an unexpected discovery. This was an acute hospital ward of mainly young men, many of whom would be going home. What kind of care they receive will depend to a large extent on whether those of us around the dying have sorted out our own death and mortality, or whether we are going to pretend death doesn't exist. Medicine is not known for its honesty—least of all over life and death issues—and the church is also struggling. Why?

9

Life and Death Issues

Since 1945 we have been living in an escapist, death-denying society. Before then the two main killers of young people were war and pneumonia. Now Europe has been at peace for over a generation, memories of Vietnam are fading, and we have penicillin and other antibiotics. These days most people assume they will live to a ripe old age. Any discussion of sickness or death is considered morbid. And now comes AIDS.

As part of a lecture on attitudes to dying I needed a photograph of a coffin. I found the mortuary attendant and an undertaker inside the hospital gates preparing to take a body outside. I asked to take a photograph of the coffin—a fibreglass box for transport to the undertakers—and they got very aggressive. They said I was sick and it was against the rules. Even though I was a doctor and the photograph was for teaching professional carers they refused. In fact I took it on the pavement outside as they were loading it into a white unmarked Ford transit van.[1]

Why the fuss? The person was unidentifiable. What is so peculiar about dying? It is just as much a part of the cycle of life as birth. The reason is that we are afraid of death. Death is the terrible unknown which robs and destroys. This fear spills over into panic, fear of illness, operations, flying, or many other things. As we will see later in this chapter, this has a profound effect on doctors and what they do.

So where are all the people who know where they are going, who have no fear of death?

You might have expected to find them in the church, but the church tends to absorb the culture of its country. The church in the West is full of this death-denying mentality. This results in a watered-down gospel promising good things now (peace, security, happincss, prosperity) because all the future rewards (heaven, eternal joy, and peace with God) have lost their meaning. People who are always talking about heaven are regarded as needing a psychiatrist—and yet that is the hope that drove the earliest Christians towards their goal. The prize St Paul was absolutely determined to win was God's call to the life above in Christ Jesus.[2] He was perfectly content to continue this life as long as God wanted because to 'live is Christ' but 'to die is gain.'[3] So what has gone wrong? If even Christians are afraid, what hope is there of dealing with the fears in the rest of our society?

The church's reaction to death

Look at the reactions of many churches to someone in their congregation who has just been told he will be dead by Christmas. The younger the congregation, the more extreme the reaction, which is why many of the rapidly growing churches are in difficulties over this whole area.

Horror

The person or his family or the church recoils with horror at the prospect of death. Having carefully put aside all thoughts about getting old, the body wearing out, and having ignored the absolute inevitability of death, the news comes as an inexplicable, unexpected disaster. The deaths of friends, colleagues, and relatives at similar ages and stages have always been written off with the philosophy of 'it will never happen to me'. The shock now produces devastation.

Frantic search for cure

Every avenue is pursued and every door pushed. Second opinions are asked for. Ever more mutilating procedures are discussed. The treating doctors often drive this madness along themselves, as a part of their own feelings of inadequacy and failure. 'Cure at all costs.'

Desperate prayers

Fear of death is what lies behind the tremendous drive towards supernatural healing in the church. Books on healing are bestsellers.[4] Healing conferences are packed. Healing meetings are standing-room only unless you arrive very early.

Within a congregation there is a drive to desperate prayers—and maybe fasting. Not the balanced prayers of faith, but the desperate prayers of fear. Gripping, overwhelming, paralysing fear of a terrible disaster. I have seen people reacting out of fear and their own emotional problems. The person they are so strenuously praying for may be totally at peace about 'going home' but others are utterly opposed to allowing events to take their natural course.

Please do not misunderstand this. I believe God heals supernaturally. I believe prayer can heal someone of AIDS and of cancer. Major healings of conditions doctors are unable to cure happen every day and I say this as a doctor. I regularly pray for people to be healed and sometimes things happen. This recent growing experience of God's healing power has gone hand in hand with a renewed emphasis on the Holy Spirit who had become a mere nebulous, ethereal 'thing' in the life and teaching of the church. The Holy Spirit is described by Jesus as the agent of his power. I am sure we are going to see far more evidence of that power over the next few years. God has given gifts and resources to the church and expects them to be used.

However the truth is that in all things God is sovereign. Who is healed and why remains a mystery. Far fewer people are healed at the moment than think they have been healed. Unless we get our fears of death sorted out we will never have a true perspective on healing.

John Wimber, well known for his work in Christian healing, before praying for a dying person will always ask: 'Is this their appointed time to die?' Wimber has no fear of death and does not necessarily see death as failure.

Confusion

Let's be honest. Usually the person is not healed. Unless you are some especially gifted person, your success rate is low with people who are terminally ill. This often leads to confusion—especially if people have been convinced that healing will or has occurred. There is a lot of unreality in the church over this which is the result of fears of death and teaching by some that God wants to heal all who are sick. Unless there is honesty, openness, and integrity, healing ministry will be brought into disrepute. If you have been healed then just as Jesus told the lepers to get their cure certified by the priests (medical experts at the time), get it checked out. Why are you so afraid of an X-ray? If God is God and he has healed you, the X-ray of your arthritis-ridden hips will be normal. If you have been healed of high blood pressure, it will be normal and remain so when (under medical supervision) the drugs are stopped.

Some conditions flare up and die down so it is hard for a doctor to certify a cure until a long time has gone by without any further episodes.

Examples are asthma, ear infections, sinusitis, epilepsy, arthritis, and AIDS. Because of the so-called placebo effect (see p. 180) many symptoms such as pain may disappear for minutes, hours or weeks simply as a result of suggestion. Yet, the disease may remain.

Questioning

The person or family may be angry: 'Why hasn't God healed me if he healed someone else in our church? Why me?' This can try the faith of the ill person, their family, and their friends.

Isolation

All too often separation occurs between those who have faith that healing has already occurred or is about to be completed, and those who are being faced with the daily reality of subtle changes in health, growing weakness, steady loss of weight, depressing blood tests, increasing pain, or shortness of breath. One group can be praying and fasting while the other is also praying but is tied up with the important process of preparing for death. This is a tragedy, especially if the latter group is tiny or non-existent apart from the ill person. If both groups are substantial, the result can be a split congregation.

Dying people tend to be chucked out of society anyway. We kid ourselves that we are caring but we are in fact rejecting. This has always been so of cancer—and has been part of the reason for hospices—and is especially so of AIDS. Apart from all the terrible fears and fantasies about touching a person who is dying with cancer (many deep down fear they can catch cancer even though they know this is irrational), there are all the intense fears of catching a plague related to AIDS.

When you don't know what to say the result may be either ludicrous conversation or oppressive awkward silence. Because both are uncomfortable, many people shy away from visiting someone who is near death or has been bereaved. If they do visit, the conversation is stilted and often meaningless to the ill person who finds entertaining his visitor exhausting. Visiting times become nightmares: the most vulnerable part of the day when literally anyone can burst onto the ward into your bedside chair and be unmovable for an hour—unless a large number of others arrive.[5]

So what is the answer to it all? The answer I believe lies in understanding the mystery of life and of death. Because nearly all my medical work is to do with those who are dying, dead, or bereaved, I am continually confronted by this issue. But there is always a first time.

'He had just left his body behind'

The first dead person I ever saw as a medical student was a huge, bloated, blue-faced man who had been pounded and punctured during a cardiac arrest. Doctors had jumped on his chest and jabbed him with needles. He came around, groaned, vomited, and died. They shocked him again, pounded him some more, sucked out the vomit, and eventually gave up. I waited and watched. Everyone drifted away. The curtains were abruptly closed off. Who was he? Who were his family? What about his wife?

I remember holding his hand and praying for him silently as he lay there, his brain gradually dying. A junior doctor came in armed with huge needles and began practising entering a vein in the neck. I asked him to stop but he refused. He carried on until he got bored and wandered out. That doctor was in charge of the patient but couldn't be bothered to find out if his wife was waiting outside. His whole attitude was cynical as though the man was merely an object, a piece of meat.[6]

I was angry and upset. How could people who had been trained to care react like this? I vowed no one I was with would ever die in such indignity.

As a Christian I believe I understood something the doctor had completely missed: a profound mystery had just taken place and I had been privileged to be present when it happened. Here was a man, a person, an individual with personality and energy, who in a moment had left this world bounded by space and time. While I watched he had just left his body behind.

Going into the dissecting room for the first time as a medical student is a strange experience. Here are people laid out on slabs, people of all shapes and sizes, distorted by long lying in formalin. Hard skin and fixed muscles. Empty shells: no one there, all long since departed. This is a mystery, the key to understanding life itself and our Creator.

That is why I count it such a privilege to look after people who are nearing the end of their lives. It is a spiritual event. The nearest an atheist gets to a religious experience is his own death, and approaching death heightens spiritual awareness in every way.

That is why deathbed conversion is so common. As we saw in an earlier chapter, Jesus welcomed the dying thief into his kingdom.[7] It seems strange that a patient who becomes a Christian in the last week of life should be loved by God in the same way as a faithful believer who has served God for decades. Jesus said that the first shall be last and the last shall be first.[8] Those who care need to look out for clues to where the person is: a newly-opened Gideon's Bible on the bedside locker, a crucifix which appears one day above the bed, a rosary in the patient's hand. These are all ways in which people tell us that things are changing inside. Sometimes conversion takes place without a word being said. A man I admitted to St Joseph's Hospice announced he was an atheist. Two weeks later he asked to see a priest. The man had undergone a radical turn-around as he approached the end.[9]

Without faith, death is the ultimate enemy; death is the robber and the destroyer. With faith in Christ, death is merely a doorway to eternity. Faith confronts us with an issue: will I enjoy eternity when I get there? Will eternity with God be heaven—or will I find eternity an unpleasant hell?

Because I have found forgiveness, inner peace, and reconciliation with God through turning to Jesus, I am looking forward to dying. While I am alive I am delighted to be allowed time here to spend with my family, building up the church, serving the community, worshipping and praising God—which is one of the most enjoyable things in my life—and telling people the good news, extending God's kingdom. However, I am just a visitor, passing through. There is nothing here which compares to what is to come. The next life is the true reality—because it is unchangeable. The earth we live on, the solar system, galaxies, space, the whole cosmos as we know it today has a very limited existence. You and I can outlive it all.

When we begin to find God's perspective on this time-space world, then death truly loses its sting. AIDS has lost its power. As doctors, the death of a patient is no longer failure but the natural transition from one existence to another. Death is not taboo any longer. We can talk about it and face up to our own mortality.

When we are with a patient who asks us if he is going to die, he can sense that we are at peace and not afraid. We can stay with him and not run away. We don't avoid spending time but are able to share experiences with him. We will not abandon him because hope of cure has abandoned us.

As a student I spent a four-week residential elective at St Christopher's Hospice. Someone said that you didn't have to have a faith to work there but those who had no faith didn't tend to last very long.

If you are a Christian I believe you have the answer. For you the mystery is understood. You know the meaning of life and the meaning of death. You understand what is happening when someone is dying. You can give meaning and hope to a person who is reaching out to God. Because Christ himself lives within you, you bring Christ to each person you meet. Every time you speak, smile, or take someone's hand, that patient comes into touch with some aspect of Christ himself.

In this book we have seen how AIDS is sweeping across the globe, leaving a terrible trail of human destruction, why the only solution in the foreseeable future is a radical change of values and human behaviour, and how failure to deal with fundamental issues like death and dying now compounds the problem of providing good care. AIDS makes us think through again our views on sexuality and life itself. It confronts us at the very root of our being and at the end of the day leaves us with choices about how we respond, not just to AIDS and those who are dying from it, but also to the ultimate issue: What is the meaning of life? What is the meaning of *my* life? Am I really just a collection of molecules, or is there another dimension?

10

An Eight-point Plan for the Government

At the end of many talks I give on AIDS, people often ask what I think the government should be doing next and what the response of churches should be. Here are some suggestions. Things are moving fast and I hope that by the time you read this, some of these decisions will already have been made.

1. Determine the extent of the problem

We need to get it right: the government does not have resources to squander on a problem that does not exist or is being exaggerated by those with vested interests in increasing their own budgets. However, we do not have time to adjust plans if the AIDS epidemic becomes worse than estimated or changes its character in any way. For example, has education reduced heterosexual spread but not affected drug addicts? Are new HIV viruses spreading in different ways? After all, as things stand, a person infected tomorrow will probably die. *You have possibly five to ten years to plan his terminal care, but only today to prevent his death.*

All discarded blood samples from selected hospital laboratories should have identifying markers removed and be sent to public health laboratories for testing. Only the hospital of origin should be stated. Results will give an indication of spread across the country and will enable us to detect local increases. Hospitals giving cause for concern should then be asked to send regular batches of blood samples with age and sex recorded on each bottle, but no other information. The United Kingdom government has recently decided to implement this proposal. Uganda has completed a full survey already.[1]

2. Target people especially at risk with further new campaigns

A prolonged, aggressive campaign needs to be aimed at the drug addict populations of major cities. They are the prime target for HIV spread in the near future. In addition, a further hard-hitting campaign needs to be aimed at all men who have had sex with other men in the past or may do so in the future—not just at the so-called gay community. Much of the momentum for change in the gay community is coming from the coffins of loved ones who have died. Multiple deaths have had a big impact in San Francisco. Government campaigns will be insufficient without continued high profile publicity for a prolonged period afterward. Education is easy. Changing behaviour is extremely difficult. Smoking kills several hundreds of thousands each year, numbers which dwarf the current AIDS problem, yet public health campaigns have taken years to produce change. Sexual drives are stronger than the power of nicotine. Only 14% of New York drug users have changed sexual behaviour, for example, while 59% are using clean needles.[2]

All educational literature should be clearly marked with date of issue and leaflets should be promptly withdrawn when out of date. There are thousands of undated leafiets printed as early as 1983 that are still circulating, perpetuating inaccurate information.

3. Get an army of health educators on the road

The economics of health education are simple: hospital costs for caring for one AIDS patient alone are so high that a health educator only has to prevent one person a year from developing AIDS to save the government or health insurance companies his entire salary.[3] If he or she succeeds in preventing one person a month from becoming infected, the government or other agencies make a fortune.

The argument for teaching prevention is overwhelming. After all, a human life is worth more than a few thousand dollars. From travelling around to schools and colleges myself, I am convinced that an effective communicator could save hundreds of lives a year.

One important factor has been left out of most school information packs and is also missing from youth education: the personal factor. It is almost useless for a teacher to spend an hour telling the facts or showing a video. Young people are bored rigid with facts. Where is the action? Who is actually dying? Is anyone dying at all? 'It's all an empty scare story. I'm not gay, so I won't get it.' When I go into a school or college everyone is on the edge of their seats. Why? Because I know people personally who have died of AIDS, people who are dying right now, and I often see people who are dying of it. It is real, so prevention and encouraging positive attitudes is easier.

The biggest asset an educator needs to have is the credibility that comes from personal experience. Even if only to be able to say he or she has visited an AIDS ward would be a tremendous help in earning the attention of students. At ACET (AIDS Care Education and Training), all our schools educators have worked in our home care programme so they have a real impact in the classroom.

A lot is being done,[4] but it is not enough. An army of health educators needs to speak to all school children over the age of eleven or twelve years.[5] It needs to happen soon. This army needs to go into colleges, universities, factories, workshops, bars, clubs, pubs, leisure centres, churches, youth groups, housing projects, community centres—anywhere people congregate. Obviously they should go in with the agreement of those in charge, but unannounced, with a high-impact, short message—'I want to tell you about three friends of mine who have just died of AIDS. I'm telling you because the person you are sitting next to right now may well be positive and all of you here in ten years' time will have been to an AIDS funeral—unless people like you listen and something changes drastically.'

4. National training programme for all health care workers

Never has there been a disease that has spread so quickly. Consider cancer care: cancer has been around for centuries and hospices for decades. Even so, there are acute training problems to keep pace with the new hospices which are opening each year. Existing units are under strain with conflicting demands from patients and from the need to train more carers.

The explosion of AIDS cases and the rapidly changing appearance of the disease—with new treatments and research likely to make most knowledge obsolete in a year or two—means that a vast, wartime-style, crash-training programme needs to be established. If each day terrorists blew up two civilian aircraft on domestic flights killing five hundred US citizens, a national state of emergency would be declared. Why shouldn't governments treat the AIDS epidemic with the same seriousness? After all, possibly twice that number are doomed each day in the United States alone through new HIV infections.

In the United States, AIDS day courses for family doctors based on voluntary attendance have had appallingly low attendance.[6] Those who come are usually those most qualified, most recently informed, and least needing the training. Where is the silent majority? Nothing but legislation will ensure that all medical personnel are effectively educated, and encouraged to have a positive attitude to AIDS patients.

An hour or half a day is totally inadequate. A full day's training should be the absolute minimum for doctors and nurses. A shorter half-day course should be compulsory after twelve to twenty-four months to provide up-to-date information on the spread of the disease and changes in management.

5. Provide a network of specialist advisory teams

Governments should fund without delay full-fledged multidisciplinary teams to advise and support health care workers in the community and various hospitals, as well as giving twenty-four-hour advice to families and friends. One aim would be to channel the latest information and techniques on treatment from research centres to those in the field. Each team should comprise an absolute minimum of one full-time doctor, two specialist nurses, a full-time social worker, and an administrator.

6. Establish a network of hostels

Governments need to slash through miles of red tape to allow the swift establishment of centrally assisted housing associations that will provide safe housing for AIDS patients who have nowhere to go, nowhere to live. Often these people are trapped in hospitals.[7] It is not unusual for a recently diagnosed person with AIDS to come back to his shared apartment and find his bags outside the door and that his partner has changed the locks. Urgent planning needs to be made for the hundreds of infected drug addicts who are appearing now in many major cities. Money needs to be released now. Failure to provide adequate care will force many onto the streets and vastly increase the spread of infection. Many will die of AIDS in the streets.

7. Recruit extra community nursing staff

AIDS patients are heavy users of nursing resources. A large group in San Francisco can only be kept out of the hospital by more or less twenty-four-hour nursing care at home. The community nursing services are already stretched to the limit by the shortened hospital stays of other patient groups, and increasing home convalescence. They are overburdened by the care of the elderly, the frail, and those who are chronically or mentally ill.

Health authorities need additional resources for community nursing that are increased automatically in line with their numbers of people with AIDS. It should not have to be renegotiated each year.

8. Fund simple remuneration of expenses for community volunteer organisations

There should be a means to remunerate the growing army of volunteer organisations for their expenses. Many volunteers for AIDS projects are giving enormous hours of help. One man has actually given up his apartment to live with a drug addict and his wife who are both dying and want to be at home.[8] Proper funding will increase this volunteer army, maintain morale, and provide extra help to professionals. Coordinating, supervising, and training volunteers professionally is a highly skilled and time-consuming job.

In addition to these points governments need to fund further major research into vaccines, cures, and better ways to prevent spread. Incentives need to be provided to encourage drug companies to direct their vast research operations towards vaccines. A comprehensive study of marriage is greatly overdue: what makes a happy marriage, how to choose the right partner, and how to prevent breakdown. Results can then be fed into schools' education programmes on AIDS, sex education, and marriage.

How can I help turn plans into action?

Letters are a very effective means of lobbying.

Petitions are useless in comparison to individual letters, so get others to write too. Write to your Member of Parliament or other appropriate government official. Even if not read, your letter will be counted as yet another part of a big vote on the issue. Write to TV producers who have made AIDS programmes. Commend them for good content and criticise the bad. Remember that in the past, thirty letters after a programme have been enough to influence the producers.

Write to your local legislators asking them what provisions they are making for those with AIDS. If you are dissatisfied with the reply, say so, and send copies of the correspondence to your newspaper.

11

A Strategy for the Church

For many, despite reading this book and listening to people speak, the first direct experience of AIDS is still going to come as a shock. This week I am wondering how to counsel someone who is planning to marry a person who may be infected. A medical colleague has recently been exposed to the virus, and I am worried that a recent illness of his could be related to AIDS. The closer to home, the harder it hits.

The church in the United Kingdom and in the United States pioneered many aspects of medical care that are taken for granted today. Almost all of the first hospitals and the associated caring agencies in England were started by Christians. Medical care was spread all over the world by a small army of dedicated men and women who often died abroad of the very diseases they went out to fight. Their living conditions were dire and primitive in Africa, Asia, South America, or China. These men and women were driven by an overwhelming compassion for those without care and without hope. For them, bringing treatment for leprosy, malaria, tuberculosis, or smallpox was bringing the love of God. As a result of that work, churches in South America, Africa, and Asia are the fastest growing in the world, at a rate enormously greater than the current birth rate. These countries are now sending missionaries to Europe and the United Kingdom, as well as to America.

Now the time has come for the church to climb off the fence, to stop taking pot-shots at the tip of the iceberg, the bit they see (erroneously) as consisting entirely of promiscuous homosexual men and drug addicts, and to start considering the whole picture: the millions of men, women and children dying worldwide. God calls us to accept all people and extend his love to them regardless of whether or not we agree with what they do.

Exploding myths

Priority number one must be to get educated. Church leaders need to be up to date and well informed. Books, conferences, and visiting speakers are all ways to achieve this. Read a paper like *The Times*, which contains excellent day-to-day reviews on what is happening. Remember that whatever you knew last year may be out of date within twelve months.

Church congregations need clear factual information about risks, about the safety of the communion cup, and about social contact. They also need clear teaching on some of the ethical issues involved. Teaching needs to be given about God's accepting love, as well as his standards, emphasising the need to care unconditionally.

Public involvement

Church leaders and their congregations need to become visibly involved. They need to be down on record, quoted in the local press, on local radio, and on record in national media, as declaring a commitment to get involved. The message is that we care about what is happening and are actively planning right now with education and training so we can be of practical assistance to the local community. Leaders especially need to come forward and to be examples—filmed talking to people with AIDS, shaking their hands, receiving communion with them, or giving them a hug. At the end of the day actions are the only things that really encourage others. Fears are not dispelled by words, but only by seeing that other people are not afraid. If church leaders cannot do this, our efforts to mobilise a congregation will become hollow.

Community care

There is a real need right now for two different kinds of support: the first is simple, basic, practical help. Typically there is someone in a hospital, maybe far from home, who really wants to go home. For various reasons this is impossible without volunteers. Maybe there are gaps in what can be provided by community services. The sort of things that are of enormous help are shopping, cooking, cleaning, mending, driving to and from hospital, gardening, walking the dog, doing the laundry, and generally being helpful.

In addition to practical help, emotional support is also needed. Sometimes the same person is able to provide both, but sometimes two different people will be needed. In San Francisco an emotional counsellor is assigned to anyone who wants one from the moment the infection is diagnosed. The purpose is to provide at least one stable caring friendship of acceptance and trust at a time of feeling intensely vulnerable, distressed, and isolated. If necessary, that person ideally is committed to continue support through all the roller-coaster ups and downs of the illness until the person dies.

Obviously there is overlap between the two kinds of help and as the person deteriorates there may be opportunities to help in other ways, for example with helping someone get washed, get to the commode, or even just get comfortable in the bed. Not everyone feels able—nor is it right for them—to give this kind of care and there should be no pressure.

Churches, or groups of churches in areas with a number of people with AIDS, are ideally placed to organise practical help and support. Such networks are growing rapidly in the United Kingdom, supported by ACET. Emotional/pastoral care will be given anyway to members of congregations with AIDS and could be extended to those outside the church according to resources. Where possible there should be the closest cooperation with other caring agencies doing similar work. Communication is a key factor to ensure good care. If in doubt communicate. Telephone is better than a letter. Communicate with family doctors, nurses, clinics, or whoever—but do not do it behind the person's back. In this way the caring network can be effective without gaps, duplication, or secrecy.

Remember that all volunteers must be carefully selected, trained, and supported. People who immediately spring to mind as ideal may turn out to be totally unsuitable. You need to find that out before they get involved rather than afterwards. Just one person can wreck your entire community programme (see Appendix B on volunteer selection).

Christian hospices

Like many other branches of medicine, hospice care was first developed by Christians. With its emphasis on allowing someone to die peacefully with dignity and respect, and on allowing people to live their last days to the full while still giving hope, it was natural that the initiative should have come almost entirely from believers. In our death-denying society, doctors and nurses drawn to this work were usually those who themselves had no fears of death, who had dealt with their own mortality because they knew by faith where they were going. Being relaxed about death and dying has been the hallmark of hospice care. Fear is infectious—but so is peace in the face of uncertainty.

Hospices are a boom industry, but almost the entire building spree is devoted to filling current gaps. Despite 1700 hospice programmes in the United States,[1] there are large areas of the country where there are no local hospice facilities for those dying of cancer who cannot be at home and who don't want to go back to hospital. Because the number of old people is increasing and we are getting better at treating other illnesses, the number of people dying of cancer is increasing each year.

As a result, hospice facilities that served an area adequately ten years ago are experiencing increasing pressure. Part of this has been relieved by the rapid development of hospice-style home care teams. However, the fact remains that cancer care alone will require the building of many more hospices by the year 2000 without any provision for people with AIDS.

Either a large number of hospices need to be planned now

for AIDS care or a large number of extra hospices need to be built accepting both cancer and AIDS patients. If this happens it could relieve pressure on existing units, allowing them to take fewer cancer patients and more people with AIDS. These decisions will continue to be influenced by community pressure. Would your relative be willing to go into a hospice which is featured on the front page of the local paper almost every week because it is now a refuge for those dying of AIDS?

Hospices have been built in the past almost entirely by local fund-raising. A number have faced near bankruptcy soon after opening. Few people appreciate that a hospice taking five years to raise a million dollars for its buildings will need a third of a million dollars each year just to keep going. In other words, the biggest fund-raising nightmare begins after it has opened when there is no longer anything visible to show for the thousands of dollars spent each month, just a few statistics of people cared for. Some hospices in the United Kingdom have had to close beds or have never been able to open fully.

In the United Kingdom, Help the Hospices is a national charity that is currently negotiating with the government to find some way out of this disaster. For the government it should make economic sense to fund most or all of the running costs—after all, the buildings are free and the cost per person per day is usually a fraction of the cost of a conventional hospital bed. However, there is only a health service saving if some hospital beds are closed to pay for the hospice. Many hospices have now successfully negotiated partial funding ranging from 30 to 60 per cent or more of annual running costs.

The AIDS crisis has thrown planners into turmoil. A hospice unit from first discussions to purchase of site, planning, design, permission, building, appointment of staff and opening usually takes three years to develop. With AIDS, the size of the problem may not have doubled, but quadrupled in four years. Yet it is difficult psychologically to start building three or four times as many hospices in 1990 as could possibly be justified in that year. It requires a huge amount of faith in statisticians. The result will be last-minute solutions: building this year to meet this year's need and next year's need. This will not allow time for prolonged fund-raising. Governments may therefore be well-disposed to partial capital funding of new ventures. Sympathy is more likely to result in government assistance if at least part of the funds have already been raised for development.

Funding for AIDS hospices will probably be less of a problem than for cancer hospices. Governments know that extra resources have to be provided. If they are not, the result will be dozens of chronically demented young people blocking acute medical and surgical beds. There are already growing pressures on hospitals to discharge these people or transfer them elsewhere. Mentally incapacitated people can be extremely hard to manage at home, particularly when accompanied by physical weakness, so pressures grow relentlessly for hospice beds.

In San Francisco, out of one hundred people with AIDS, over twenty will be in a bed somewhere. The rest will be at home. Ten will be in an acute ward with, for example, a new chest infection, and the other ten will require chronic twenty-four-hour nursing care. To provide this level of care at home is far more expensive than in a hospice. At home the ratio of nurse to patient is one to one. In a hospice the same nurse can look after several people. If only intermittent nursing is required the costs shift in favour of home care, especially if volunteers are used from an agency like ACET. The average stay in a chronic care unit is between two and four months.

If a group of churches or individuals are interested in exploring a local hospice initiative, further guidelines are given in Appendix A.

You may be an individual reading this and wanting to get involved somehow. I suggest the following:

- Talk to your church leader/minister. He may be aware of new local initiatives. He may also be able to give some helpful advice.
- In the absence of any local church response consider becoming involved in a secular group helping those with AIDS. Explain where you live, and that you would like to offer practical help. You will probably be asked to go through a selection

and training session. Get involved, be helpful.

- Keep your eyes open for new local church initiatives. With your training and experience you could be an invaluable resource to a new pastoral counselling project, a new volunteer agency, or a new hospice.
- Keep in touch with your own church so they know what you are up to and can support you and pray for you. Educate the church so it is ready for people with AIDS to be a part of the fellowship.
- Remember you are a servant. You are not there for any other reason. If you have any other motives at all, do not get involved. If you want to evangelise the world, go and evangelise the world, but don't regard the volunteer programme as your pitch to get at AIDS patients, their friends, or their families.

True care involves accepting the person you care for on that person's own terms. You may have a different outlook, different perspectives, different beliefs, different views on personal behaviour, but these need to be laid to one side. You do not have to agree in order to care, but you do need to respect the person and not seek to impose your own perspectives on the one you are caring for.

12

What you can do about AIDS

As a result of reading this book you may be wondering what you should do about AIDS. Here are various practical things you can do depending on your own situation.

1. Worried about infection

If you are concerned about contracting AIDS, the first thing you should do is change your lifestyle: have one partner (currently uninfected) for life and do not inject drugs.

If you are a heterosexual, living in the West and not injecting drugs, the risk that you could be infected is very small unless you have been taking risks in the last four years. People are often worried about things they were doing in the late 1970s or early 1980s. Almost all those infected during that time were gay or bisexual men.

You may feel you have good reasons to be worried. You need expert advice from a physician with experience in this area as a result of which you may want to be tested. You need to think this through carefully. The decision to be tested is not straightforward and you need good preparation if you decide to go ahead. If the test comes back positive things can happen very fast. In the upset you can end up sharing the result with someone who then lets you down by telling other people. The result can be a lost job or worse, so you need to have thought through what you will do if the result if positive.

You may have been required under state law to have a test because you are about to get married. Many people are choosing to get married somewhere else to avoid a test. But this is one area where testing is especially important: here are two people committing themselves to each other for life and probably intending to have a family. I know people who have decided to be tested because of their past lives, out of courtesy and respect for a future spouse.

2. Living with a postive test

A positive test result needs checking a second time to be absolutely sure. The result can occasionally be wrong. A confirmed positive result means your body has been exposed to the virus. Some of your soldier cells will have been reprogrammed. We have to make sure that those soldier cells stay asleep for as long as possible before being stimulated by other infections into producing more virus particles.

Anything that would improve the health of an uninfected person is also likely to give the very best chance of health to someone who is infected. Boosting your immune system will also help your body keep well if some of your soldier cells are starting to die.[1]

Eat a balanced diet, avoid physical exhaustion, and pace yourself in what you do. Exercise regularly and be careful about situations you know are likely to leave you completely drained emotionally. It seems that some people can live for many years—even decades—with this virus. The longer you live, the more likely it is that we will find more effective treatments or even a cure.

A lot of people may try to exploit your fears by selling you all kinds of treatments or remedies. Before you spend your savings on these things, just remember that every drug company in the world would love to find a natural substance that could work well for people with AIDS. Every folk remedy you hear about has already been examined and rejected by scientists or is as yet unproven. Most of these things gain their reputation because people who take them often seem to improve. However, as we have seen, what makes people with AIDS ill is usually the other infections that invade when the soldier cells are damaged. The natural course of the illness can be a series of dramatic ups and downs. People then credit a folk remedy for an improvement that was bound to happen anyway.

I do not want to stop you from trying these things but many people have wasted a lot of money on 'cures' that are totally worthless.[2]

3. First signs of becoming ill

You may panic because, having read this book, you think you are suffering from the early stages of AIDS. This illness is a great mimic of other less serious conditions. For example, a fever together with swollen glands for a while is quite likely to be caused by glandular fever. All kinds of things can produce rashes or diarrhoea. If you are worried, you should see a physician.

However, you may know that you are a carrier of the virus, and your physician has confirmed that the virus is now making you ill. Exactly the same things apply as for those infected but feeling well: basically, take care of your body to give it the best environment to protect you.

4. Full-blown AIDS

If you are infected with AIDS, you have probably already become an expert on the disease. Some days you may feel able to handle it and other days you may feel you are not coping at all. However you became infected, and whatever your background, not far from where you live there are other people in the same situation who may be able to help you. AIDS is too big a burden for anyone to have to carry on his or her own. Sometimes you will find yourself caught between facing the practicalities of dying and wanting to build plans for the next two decades.

Whatever your situation, there are a number of agencies available to help you practically, emotionally, and spiritually. They are listed at the back of this book.

5. Partner infected or ill

Often it is more harrowing to watch someone else suffering than to be in the situation yourself. You can feel helpless and frustrated. On top of all that can be the exhaustion that comes from giving care twenty-four hours a day, seven days a week.

There can also be a lurking unease that your partner may have infected you or that you infected your partner. All these things can produce high levels of anxiety and stress.

Again I urge you to link up with all the available agencies for practical and emotional support. You may be encouraged to know that many partners have not infected each other even after long periods of unprotected sex. You will need to think through that whole area now in the light of the chapter in this book about condoms and the advice to partners of infected people.

6. Wanting to set up a volunteer programme

There is a real need right now for a national network of volunteers to provide practical help at home for those with AIDS. The organisation I began, AIDS Care Education and Training (ACET), is a church-based care project in the United Kingdom. Churches in other countries have a vitally important part to play too. But when starting a volunteer programme, several factors need to be kept in mind to ensure its success and effectiveness.

How to start a volunteer programme

An organisation run entirely by volunteers should be just as professional and twice as well-organised as a hospice. Co-ordinating offers of availability without producing chaos requires great skill, dedication, and hard work.

Selection

Careful selection of volunteer workers is essential. In the United Kingdom we have found a questionnaire to all would-be volunteers is helpful. What motivates them? Are they seeking this position to work out problems of their own? Guilt? Confused sexuality? Homophobia? Recent unresolved grief? Do they think they might be infected themselves? What are they hoping to achieve? What will they find most rewarding? What will they find most difficult?

Someone I know said to me that all she wanted to do was to

'get onto an AIDS ward and tell everyone about Jesus'. The trouble is that if she found her way into a volunteer programme (as she might if the selection procedures are sloppy), in five minutes she could destroy five years of goodwill, making it almost impossible for any Christian organisation to continue working in that area.

People are sensitive, and rightly so, to someone coming in and 'Bible-bashing'. It takes only one insensitive, over-zealous person to damage a whole organisation. There is a right time and a right place.

The important thing is to be a servant; if someone asks you why you are doing what you are doing, there may well be opportunity to share the hope that is in you. However, you are crazy if you think a medical agency is going to refer people with AIDS to you for help when they find out that you abuse that position of trust by preaching or moralising. You will destroy the credibility of your service. As a volunteer, your behaviour should be just as professional as if you were a hospital doctor.

References from employers, ministers, or church leaders are important. All these things can form the basis of an interview. Reliability is absolutely essential.

Training

Most people with AIDS are well-informed about their condition—they have to be with so much misinformation and ignorance around.

It is rude, insensitive, and unfair to send in a volunteer who is ignorant about the disease. Training should include not only clear factual presentations but also opportunity for people to work through hidden reactions to homosexuality, fear of dying, and fear of disease. These sessions should be part of the final selection process and no one should be accepted as a volunteer before completing this training. One-to-one counselling may also be necessary following a training session and, if in a church context, pastoral help and prayer.

Support

A useful part of the training programme is developing friendships between volunteers and existing team members. The work is stressful. It can be harrowing to visit someone a few hours from death and spend time with them as they pour out their anger against the impotence of doctors' false promises, dead hopes, and dashed aspirations. It can be hard to stay with someone who keeps asking, 'Why me?' It can be distressing to be with a dying person and to leave them knowing they may then die alone. Support is essential: a network of caring friendships between like-minded people who have experienced the same things and can understand. If you are part of a church, make sure that a few people you trust know what you are doing so they can support and pray for you.

What sort of things can volunteers to?

This depends on experience, personality, and availability. Each volunteer has special potential which needs to be harnessed creatively. A retired nurse provides a different type of help from that of an out-of-work builder.

Shopping, laundry, gardening, cleaning, cooking, walking the dog, mending things around the house, driving a person to and from clinics, and being a friend are important ways to serve any sick person. A good attitude is that of a servant. Basically say, 'I am here. I am available now and at these times in the future. What can I do that would be helpful?' Then suggest some things that you would be willing and able to do. Sometimes it is helpful just to have a volunteer sit in the home to allow a friend or relative to go out. The main caregiver can feel trapped—unable to leave the room or the house with a sick person needing constant attention. After a while exhaustion sets in.

There should be a central place where volunteers report after a visit to be given up-to-date information. A coordinator should be able to spot a volunteer who is getting out of his/her depth or is becoming over-involved to the detriment of personal well-being.

Seven basic rules for volunteers

1. Communicate frequently with others.
2. Always be utterly reliable and punctual.
3. Respect privacy of the person you are visiting. It is his/her life and home.
4. Remember that touch is important and a hug can mean more than a thousand words.
5. Be sensitive to the needs of the patient.
6. Be careful not to overstay your welcome.
7. Be a servant, caring unconditionally in a non-judgemental way.

It may be especially helpful if volunteers are attached to a medical support team or to a local hospice. This ensures proper supervision and medical back-up.

7. Wanting to prevent infection

Education means persuading people to change behaviour so they are no longer taking risks, or risks are enormously reduced. The most effective persuaders are those who can talk from the heart and not just from the head. People whose own lives have been affected as partners, friends, people with AIDS, or as home care volunteers have the greatest impact. You need to do all you can to ensure such people have good access into schools, colleges, factories, bars, and clubs to talk with those as yet untouched. This will be much more effective than advertising alone. As we have seen, an educator only needs to prevent one infection a year to save his government his entire salary in treatment and hospital bills alone.

The future of your own country is in your hands. You can write, phone, or otherwise make your views known to those in local or national government, to health planners, and to church leaders. You can make sure copies of this book get to the right people—all profits go to an AIDS charity. You may feel that your contribution is small and not worth much, but thousands of others are doing the same. Together we can help turn the tide and build a better place for those who come after us. We are too late to prevent a disaster but not too late to prevent an even bigger one.

APPENDICES

APPENDIX A

Hospice, hospital, or home?

AIDS is not like cancer. As we have seen, people with AIDS can be acutely ill of pneumonia, need intensive care, recover, and go home. Such people need to be in acute hospital wards with access to all laboratory facilities. They need X-rays as well as a vast variety of special procedures and tests using very expensive and specialised equipment. Fluid may need to be taken from the lungs, spine, or abdomen in order to find out what antibiotic to use.

Hospices cannot provide this except at vast expense. Some places could be half-way houses offering the best of both: In the United Kingdom, the Mildmay, for example, has a fully equipped operating theatre, X-ray department, clinic areas, and other things in addition to its beautiful new hospice-style, single-roomed ward with roof-top gardens. AIDS patients could be managed at Mildmay from diagnosis to death.

There are three other groups of people, however, not requiring quick access to intensive care facilities. The first are people who have already been through two or three awful pneumonias and have decided that the next time they want to die peacefully without several days of tubes everywhere, fighting for every breath. They know they are going to die and they are so tired, so thin and wasted, that they are ready to think about a hospice. The second group of people is where the virus has caused cancer, usually Kaposi's sarcoma, the blue skin tumour—and cancer is their main problem. These people could be admitted to cancer hospices. The third group is made up of people whose brain cells have been attacked by the AIDS virus and who are slowly losing their memory and independence. These people often require an enormous amount of nursing care in addition to support for patient, friends, and family. They do not require intensive care. A hospice may be ideal.

If they had the choice, most people would prefer to die in their own homes. The main reason people choose not to is because they feel unsafe and afraid of what might happen at home. Friends or family may also find it hard to cope. Cancer home care support teams, many of which are attached to hospices, are increasingly willing to help people with AIDS. However, these teams either need rapid expansion in certain areas to manage the extra workload or new specialist teams need to be set up.

New specialist teams are only practical in areas with large numbers of suitable AIDS patients. The big argument in their favour is that they could get involved in the pre-AIDS situation if necessary and certainly with their specialised knowledge they could enable someone in the acute stages with pneumocystis pneumonia to be treated successfully at home. A cancer team is really geared to manage a chronically deteriorating patient in his or her last weeks. Volunteer-based groups can fill a useful gap in areas where there are not enough people with AIDS to justify specialist medical teams.

In summary, the right place for someone to be at any time is where they want to be. We must provide options for people to choose for themselves. Options allow someone to keep control over his or her own life and live with dignity and self-respect even while losing independence in other ways.

As Dame Cicely Saunders, pioneer of Hospice Care, once said, 'The aim is to help someone to live fully until he or she dies.'

APPENDIX B

Burnout among AIDS Care Workers —How it Spot it, How to Avoid it

'Burnout' is a loose term used to describe what happens to some people in the caring profession when they have given out too much for too long, have become too drained and have been lacking support, quality time off, and opportunity for understanding.[1]

It starts when a warm caring person begins to distance himself or herself from people, in order to gain protection from further suffering. The person may become profoundly depressed, bursting into tears for little apparent reason, taking time off work, sleeping badly, not coping at all. Overinvolvement is another danger sign. When a volunteer is asked to go in from 10.30 to 12.30 to help with housework but regularly stays at the home until 11.00pm, I would say that volunteer is a good candidate for burnout.

Now there are times when we all switch off. But if I burst into tears at the scene of a major car accident I would not be much use as a doctor. As a medical student I used to feel faint at the sight of blood and sometimes I still do, but I have to harden myself in order to get a job done. Nor are we emotionally capable of identifying fully with every person's suffering. Jesus was able to—and is able to now—but we are more limited. Dame Cicely Saunders, founder of St Christopher's Hospice, once said that the most important thing you can ever give your patient is your tears and the knowledge that you will miss him when he is gone. That is true. Tears are a part of my life as a member of a support team and a part of my life as a member of a team of leaders in my church. If we cannot laugh and don't know how to cry then what are we made of? The shortest verse in the Bible is this: 'Jesus wept.'[2] He was grief-stricken.

However, there are times when I need someone to point out danger areas. I remember when working at St Joseph's Hospice in Hackney, I was looking after a young woman who had shown great courage over many months with pain that was sometimes very hard to relieve. After much suffering she developed a pneumonia. I prescribed antibiotics and was confronted by the ward sister whom I respected enormously. She felt strongly that I had made the wrong decision. I backed down only after the intervention of a senior medical colleague. Eventually I realised that I was too emotionally involved with this patient to be capable of any rational decisions regarding her treatment.

The patient was a very strong character who had often been hard for us to care for but over time I grew fond of her. Having wished sometimes that her suffering would end, I now found myself unable to let go and let her die.[3]

In actual fact, as in so many of these things, I do not think antibiotics would have made any difference—she was very near death and deteriorating rapidly. I found the whole thing very distressing. Now if that sort of thing was happening two or three times a week, you can see that in a month or two I would become emotional jelly. Should I have not cared about her? Not at all. But let us care for each other, care for the caregivers, listen to each other, protect each other, and share the load.

Support teams crack up and pack up with monotonous regularity due to lack of care and personality clashes. Together we can avoid these things.

APPENDIX C

Advice to Travellers Going Abroad

Be extremely careful when abroad to make sure that you receive no untested blood, contaminated injections, or blood tests with re-used needles. In some areas up to one in five of all units of blood provided by hospitals may be infected.

Try at all costs to avoid being compulsorily tested for AIDS by a developing country as part of its screening of long-stay visitors. AIDS tests can be wrongly done and can give false positive results. The consequences for you could be terrible.

Some countries now require a negative blood test certificate for certain groups of people to enter. Many countries refuse entry to someone with AIDS or people who are positive.

People travelling abroad should be warned that in many major cities of the world, half of all prostitutes are now positive. Infection rates are also likely to be high in men or women who hang around bars and clubs and have a promiscuous lifestyle. A recent report estimated that heterosexual residents of the United Kingdom are three hundred times more at risk each week they spend in another country than they are at home.[1]

TRAVEL RESTRICTIONS ON HIV-INFECTED PERSONS

This is a summary of proposed and existing travel restrictions as far as can be ascertained from enquiries of embassies and consulates in London. HIV-Ab^+ = antibody positive; HIV-Ab^- = antibody negative.

Country	Type of visitor	Type of restriction
Algeria	Students from sub-Saharan Africa	Tested on arrival.
Australia	Compulsory HIV testing for permanent resident applicants over 15 years old and children under 15 who have had a blood transfusion, show symptoms of AIDS or are to be adopted by Australian residents. Temporary residence, tourist or other short-term visa applicants are excluded	
Austria (Klagenfurt only)	Foreign workers applying for a residence permit	Must be certified HIV-Ab^-.
Belgium	Foreign students applying for Belgian Government scholarships	Compulsory testing in country of origin.
Belize	Foreign workers or migrants	Certified HIV-Ab^- not more than 3 months earlier.

Bulgaria	Foreign nationals staying more than 1 month; for British students an Ab^- certificate obtained in the UK is an option	Compulsory testing within 15–20 days of arrival.
Cambodia	Visa applicants must provide an HIV negative certificate. However, enforcement of this requirement is uneven	Certified HIV-Ab^-.
Chile	Unspecified HIV entry requirements under consideration. Foreigners staying over 3 months require a general health certificate from a doctor—HIV not specified	
China, People's Republic of	Foreigners staying over 1 year (some sources suggest 6 months but this has not been confirmed), and permanent resident applicants. Diplomats are exempt	HIV-Ab test in UK must be approved by Chinese Embassy or Consulate.
Colombia	Visitors from USA, Haiti, and Africa (under consideration)	Certified HIV-Ab^-.
Costa Rica	Foreign nationals staying more than 3 months	Tested on arrival.
Cuba	Foreign workers and overseas students, long-term foreign residents and Cubans returning from endemic areas	Tested on arrival.

Country	Type of visitor	Type of restriction
Cyprus	Foreign nationals seeking work permits to work in nightclubs or as cabaret artists. All African students. Long-term residence visa applicants	Tested on arrival.
Czechoslovakia	Foreign students and resident workers from countries with high HIV rates	Compulsory testing on arrival. HIV-Ab^{+} repatriated.
Egypt	Foreign contractors entering Egyptian military facilities, and those working for more than one month	
Finland	Foreign workers	Screening to be introduced.
France	HIV testing is not required for an alien residence card. However, applicants with clinical symptoms of AIDS may be tested and, if found seropositive, may be denied a residence card	HIV-Ab^{+} may be denied card.
Germany	Applicants for a resident permit more than 90 days. Exemptions: EEC nationals; nationals of Andorra, Finland, Iceland, Liechtenstein, Malta, Monaco, Norway, Austria, San Marino, Sweden, Switzerland, Vatican City. Students receiving scholarships from Ministry of Economic Co-operation	Compulsory testing.

Germany (East)	Foreigners staying in GDR or East Berlin for more than 3 months. Diplomats exempt	HIV-AB$^-$ or screened on arrival.
Greece	Foreign students studying under Greek government scholarship and foreign performing artists planning to work in Greece	Compulsory testing.
Hungary	No requirements at present. Testing perhaps if HIV infection is suspected	
India	Overseas students and foreigners staying more than 1 year (except diplomats, journalists, and subjects under 18 years).	Compulsory testing within 1 month of arrival.
Indonesia	Visitors suspected of having AIDS or being HIV-Ab$^-$	Refused entry.
Iraq	Overseas visitors staying over 5 days (except diplomats, children less than 12 years and adults more than 65 years), British nationals	Compulsory testing within 5 days of arrival at specified clinics/hospitals, HIV-Ab$^-$ certificate obtained in UK option.
Japan	On December 23, 1988, the Japanese Diet approved an AIDS prevention bill which bars entry of HIV-infected foreigners and authorises mandatory HIV testing of suspected HIV-infected individuals or AIDS patients seeking entry into Japan	Only tested if suspected HIV infected.

Country	Type of visitor	Type of restriction
Korea (North)	Foreign nationals, researchers, students, trainees and athletes staying over 91 days require HIV negative certificates issued one month before arrival. Foreign diplomats (and families), journalists, clergymen and US soldiers are exempt. Implementation date unknown	Certified HIV-Ab^-, or else submit to mandatory HIV test within 72 hours of arrival.
Kuwait	Foreign nationals applying for residence permits for longer than 6 months	Must be certified HIV-Ab^-.
Libya	Foreign workers, long-term visitors and residence applicants. Official delegations and visitors are exempt.	Must be certified HIV-Ab^-.
Malaysia	Foreign nationals suspected of having HIV infection—not tourists	Tested on arrival.
Mongolia	Overseas students (Own needles may be used.) Tests repeated several months later	May be tested on arrival.
Nigeria	Nationals of any country that introduces mandatory HIV screening for Nigerian travellers	

Pakistan	Foreigners staying more than one year need to provide a negative HIV certificate when applying for a visa in the UK. Those not in possession will be tested in Pakistan at a designated laboratory. Foreign diplomats are exempt.	
Philippines	All immigrants, refugees, illegal residents, visitors for longer than 6 months, all foreign sailors and aliens seeking a change from temporary to permanent resident. US military personnel and US government civilian employees are exempt	Tested.
Poland	Foreign students may be tested	
Qatar	Foreign work permit applicants and foreign students. Diplomats are exempt	Compulsory testing.
Saudi Arabia	Work permit applicants. Retesting after 3 months residence is now required of all foreign workers. Families are exempt	Must be certified HIV-Ab^-.
Singapore	Foreign maids tested before entry. Foreigners who are HIV-Ab^+ are repatriated	
South Africa	Foreign workers (not generally European workers)	Compulsory testing.

Country	Type of visitor	Type of restriction
Sri Lanka	Foreign nationals suspected of having HIV infection	May be refused entry or deported.
Syria	Foreign nationals applying for work permits and foreign students	Compulsory testing on arrival, at specified centres. British nationals may provide certificate.
Taiwan	Foreign students from 'epidemic areas'	Must be certified HIV-Ab^-.
Thailand	Foreign nationals known to have AIDS or HIV infection	Refused entry.
Turkey	The health ministry reported in April 1988 that 75 centres have been established, mainly at border checkpoints and tourism areas, to conduct HIV screening tests. However no formal testing requirement has been published.	
United Arab Emirates	Foreigners applying for work or residence permits or permit renewals or foreigners staying more than 30 days. Diplomats are exempt	Compulsory testing.
United Kingdom	Visitors suspected of having AIDS in need of extensive medical treatment	May be refused entry.

Union of Soviet Socialist Republics (USSR)	Foreign nationals over 15 years old staying more than 3 months. Foreigners leaving the USSR, returning after 1 month and staying more than 3 months must produce a new certificate not more than 1 month old	Compulsory testing on arrival; or certified HIV-Ab^- within previous 30 days. Compulsory testing. HIV-Ab^- refused entry.
United States of America	Applicants for immigrant visas, refugees, and aliens seeking permanent residence	Compulsory testing.
Venezuela	Foreign visitors (under consideration)	Certified HIV–HIV-Ab^-.
Vietnam	Refugees returning from Hong Kong will be tested	

Reprinted by kind permission of the Bureau of Hygiene and Tropical Diseases, Keppel Street, London WC1E 7HT. Tel: 071-636 8636.

APPENDIX D

Checklist of Countries[1]

Some people still think that you can only get infected with HIV if you are in the United States, United Kingdom, or Africa. However, almost every country in the world is affected. The update of these figures since the first edition in August 1987 has been an alarming and depressing task. African countries are reporting huge increases as are those in Western Europe. Figures in Western Europe have increased slightly more slowly than predicted in 1987.

Please note that the following figures show only those cases of full-blown AIDS reported up to May 1990. Figures are in reality often much higher due to unwillingness of governments to admit the extent of the problem, and failure of each government's information agencies to hear about many who have died. Numbers in themselves do not reflect the size of the problem in any country, and need to be seen in the context of the size of the country. The Bahamas, for example, have only reported four hundred and thirty-seven cases. However, its total population is tiny, indicating an average of eighty cases per one hundred thousand people. In contrast, Australia reports nearly five times as many cases (1789), but because its population is nearly sixteen million people, the number of cases per one hundred thousand is less than four. Remember to multiply any estimate by ten to give total numbers of people who are actually ill (early disease).

World Health Organisation reports in May 1990 indicate the following:

Global total AIDS reports: 254,078 (April 1990)

60% heterosexual
15% homosexual
10% mother to baby
10% drug injecting
5% blood products/transfusion

Dr James Chin, Head of Surveillance Forecasting at WHO, estimates that within 10 years, AIDS will be the leading cause of death among young and middle aged adults in urban North America and sub-Saharan Africa. He sees young adult mortality rates quadrupling in these areas.

World Health Organisation estimates for infection have been set at the absolute bottom end of the possible range and are as follows:

Africa:	5.0 million
Europe:	0.5 million
Americas:	2.5 million
Asia:	0.5 million

He estimates total world infection of 15–20 million people by the year 2000 with six million cases of AIDS. WHO now expect only half those infected to develop AIDS in 10 years, 75% in 15 years and possibly all to develop AIDS after 20 years.[2] These are longer than estimates made two years ago, and mean there will be an even longer delay between behaviour changes and any effect on illness rates. AIDS deaths will leave ten million orphans by the year 2000.

Western Europe	No. cases	Date of Report
1. Austria	415	March 31, 1990
2. Belgium	596	December 31, 1989
3. Cyprus	15	February 15, 1990
4. Denmark	573	March 31, 1990
5. Finland	58	March 31, 1990
6. France	8.883	December 31, 1989. Highest number of cases in Europe. Deaths by 1991–92 are expected to exceed road deaths. Public dismisses it as a gay problem. In Paris the majority of new infections are in heterosexuals.
7. West Germany	4,653	March 31, 1990. Numbers are doubling every eighteen months, 37,816 cases of HIV infection recorded.
8. Greece	295	March 31, 1990.
9. Greenland		First infected person in October 1985. No full-blown cases of AIDS (March 31, 1987).
10. Iceland	13	March 31, 1990.
11. Ireland	124	December 31, 1990.
12. Italy	6,068	March 31, 1990. Numbers are doubling every 8–12 months.
13. Luxembourg	24	December 31, 1990
14. Malta	14	December 31, 1990.
15. Netherlands	1,189	March 31, 1990. Intensive campaign to educate drug addicts.
16. Norway	153	March 31, 1990.
17. Portugal	410	March 31, 1990.
18. Spain	5,295	March 31, 1990. Six out of ten drug addicts

			and seven out of ten haemophiliacs are positive; two out of three cases are in drug users.
19.	Sweden	380	December 31, 1989. Positive people can be put in prison by law if they continue unsafe sex.
20.	Switzerland	1,255	March 31, 1990. Because these are in a small population, Switzerland has the highest per capita number of AIDS cases in Europe.
21.	United Kingdom	3,247	April 30, 1990. Numbers were doubling every eighteen months. Estimates ranged from twenty thousand to forty thousand of numbers infected.

Eastern Europe

1.	Albania	No	cases by December 31, 1989.
2.	Bulgaria	7	June 30, 1988. But massive health education and screening.
3.	Czechoslovakia	23	March 31, 1990.
4.	East Germany	19	December 31, 1989.
5.	Hungary	34	March 31, 1990.
6.	Poland	35	March 31, 1990.
7.	Romania	74	February 8, 1990. Hundreds of young children infected through micro-transfusions and dirty needles.
8.	USSR	26	January 15, 1990. Homosexuality and drug abuse have always been denied as problems until recently. A paper was presented a few months ago on a large group of people suffering from a rare kind of cancer—it was, of course, Kaposi's sarcoma. It told us that the USSR almost certainly has a major problem. Condoms are virtually unobtainable, and promiscuity/drug abuse abound. A recent report[3] shows 102 people out of a million tested were infected. If this was the situation in the whole country, that would give a total of infected people of around thirty thousand. Minister of Health estimates 1.5 million people in the USSR will be infected by the year 2000.
9.	Yugoslavia	120	March 31, 1990.

North America

1.	United States	126,127	April 11, 1990.
2.	Canada	3,735	April 2, 1990.

Oceania

1.	Australia	1,789	March 23, 1990 and doubling every two years. A BBC report in early 1987 claimed the problem was growing faster in Australia than anywhere outside Africa.
2.	French Polynesia	13	January 20, 1990; 130 infected people identified.
3.	New Zealand	156	January 11, 1990.

North Africa and Middle East

Islamic countries forbid homosexuality. Drug abuse is rarely acknowledged.

1.	Algeria	13	March 26, 1990.
2.	Bahrain	No	cases by February 15, 1990.
3.	Egypt	16	February 15, 1990.
4.	Iran	9	February 15, 1990.
5.	Iraq	No	cases by February 15, 1990.
6.	Israel	109	March 31, 1990.
7.	Jordan	9	February 15, 1990.
8.	Kuwait	1	February 15, 1990.
9.	Lebanon	31	February 15, 1990.
10.	Libya	No	cases by February 15, 1990.
11.	Morocco	45	January 31, 1990.
12.	Oman	14	February 15, 1990.
13.	Saudi Arabia	6	cases from blood transfusions by December 31, 1988.
14.	Syria	8	February 15, 1990.
15.	Tunisia	50	February 15, 1990.
16.	Turkey	31	January 31, 1990.
17.	United Arab Emirates	1	case and 70 known to be infected by March 31, 1987.
18.	Yemen	No	cases by December 31, 1988.
19.	Peoples Democratic Republic of Yemen	No	cases by February 15, 1990.

Africa

The World Health Organisation estimates at least 3.5 million are infected. However, since good data from Uganda indicate 1 million infected there out of only 8 million adults, and other neighbouring countries are also badly affected, it seems likely that the WHO estimate is very conservative. The truer figure could be more than 7 million. These figures are what governments are officially willing to admit and bear no resemblance to the size of the disaster. Women are more frequently affected than men, and many of their children are infected or later orphaned. Rates of infection outside towns and cities seem to be lower.

1. Angola	104	December 31, 1988.
2. Benin	60	September 5, 1989.
3. Botswana	87	January 17, 1990.
4. Burundi	2,784	December 31, 1989.
5. Cameroon	78	March 31, 1989. One in one hundred of all hospital patients (non-AIDS) tested positive. Eight out of one hundred prostitutes were positive.
6. Central African Republic	662	December 31, 1989. Eight out of one hundred of population positive. Two out of ten prostitutes positive.
7. Chad	21	November 17, 1989.
8. Congo	1,250	December 8, 1988. Five out of one hundred of population (in town) positive. With fifteen to twenty cases per week at one hospital alone (25 per cent of all beds are AIDS-related). Shortages of needles and condoms.
9. Ethiopia	348	February 28, 1990.
10. Gambia	81	March 8, 1990.
11. Ghana	1,240	January 31, 1990.
12. Ivory Coast	3,647	February 1, 1990.
13. Kenya	6,004	July 30, 1989. 50 per cent Nairobi prostitutes infected. Up to 90 per cent prostitutes infected in some areas; and 1–2 per cent of all blood transfusions infected. Testing facilities inadequate in 1988. 60 per cent of AIDS cases in western part of country.[4]
14. Lesotho	8	September 15, 1989.
15. Malawi	7,160	January 8, 1990. One hospital reported 100% seropositivity in pregnant women.
16. Mali	178	October 31, 1990.
17. Mozambique	84	March 20, 1990.

18. Nigeria	35	August 2, 1989. Amazing considering eight out of one hundred tested in Lagos were infected in 1988. One local report expects numbers to rise to 1,200 with 1.2 million infected.
19. Rwanda	2,285	December 31, 1989. Eighteen out of one hundred blood donors are positive in Kigali. One report of 16 per cent of those tested infected. Extensive education campaign.
20. South Africa	353	February 15, 1990. 6% of newborn babies infected in Soweto. Numbers doubling every 8–12 months.
21. Swaziland	14	June 16, 1988.
22. Tanzania	6,251	March 1, 1990. Four out of ten barmaids were positive, one in ten blood donors in Dar es Salaam, and seven out of one hundred of the general population in Musonia were positive.
23. Tunisia	50	February 15, 1990.
24. Uganda	12,444	December 31, 1989. Eleven out of one hundred blood donors are infected in Kampala, fourteen out of one hundred pregnant women, and over a third of all patients attending hospitals in Kampala and Masaka, are all infected (some reports). One in eight of all adults (1 million) estimated infected in 1990.
25. Zaire	11,732	January 31, 1990. But around seven out of one hundred of all adult patients in Kinshasa are infected. Fourteen out of one hundred children four years old and under, are infected too. People with AIDS at one Kinshasa hospital were being sent home to die as soon as the disease was diagnosed. Otherwise the hospital would have had to close.
26. Zambia	2,709	January 29, 1990. Eight out of one hundred people examined in routine check-ups in Lusaka are infected. Six thousand infected babies were expected in 1987.[5] Fifteen out of one hundred blood donors give infected blood. In May 1986 the government banned all doctors from giving any information about AIDS. All information is now issued by the government.

27. Zimbabwe	2,357	March 31, 1990. But some sources say one in ten young people infected in some areas, and many deaths are reported. Estimated two hundred and fifty thousand infected in 1987. Unconfirmed reports of 60% of armed forces infected.

Central and South America

1. Argentina	566	December 31, 1989.
2. Belize	11	September 30, 1988.
3. Bolivia	11	June 30, 1989.
4. Brazil	10,510	March 30, 1990. Spreading rapidly through prostitution, blood transfusions, drug abuse. The majority are not homosexuals. Official estimates of one hundred and twenty thousand infected people.
5. Chile	178	December 31, 1989.
6. Colombia	643	December 31, 1989.
7. Costa Rica	151	December 31, 1989.
8. Ecuador	72	September 9, 1989.
9. El Salvador	165	December 31, 1989.
10. French Guiana	150	June 30, 1989.
11. Guatemala	65	December 31, 1989.
12. Guyana	84	December 31, 1989.
13. Honduras	512	December 31, 1989.
14. Mexico	4,131	April 20, 1990.
15. Nicaragua	4	December 31, 1989.
16. Panama	180	December 31, 1989.
17. Paraguay	13	September 30, 1989.
18. Peru	254	December 31, 1989.
19. Suriname	48	December 31, 1989.
20. Uruguay	90	March 31, 1990.
21. Venezuela	646	September 30, 1989. But between two and three out of one hundred of the entire population may be infected according to recent random testing.

Caribbean

1. Anguilla	4	December 31, 1989.
2. Antigua	3	June 30, 1988.

3. Bahamas	437	December 31, 1989. Six in every one thousand blood donors are infected.
4. Barbados	112	December 31, 1989.
5. British Virgin Islands	1	September 30, 1989.
6. Bermuda	135	December 31, 1989.
7. Cayman Islands	5	September 30, 1989.
8. Cuba	63	June 30, 1988.
9. Dominica	10	December 31, 1989.
10. Dominican Republic	1,200	December 31, 1989. One in one hundred blood donors is infected.
11. Grenada	19	February 28, 1990.
12. Guadeloupe	175	November 13, 1989.
13. Haiti	2,331	September 30, 1989. Nearly one in ten men emigrating to Florida is infected. Six out of one hundred mothers with young children are positive. The problem is fifty to one hundred times as bad as in Europe – similar to Africa.
14. Jamaica	141	February 28, 1990.
15. Martinique	115	December 31, 1989.
16. Montserrat	1	June 30, 1989.
17. Puerto Rico	312	March 31, 1987. Four out of ten are not drug addicts or homosexuals.
18. St Christopher's and Nevis	18	December 31, 1988.
19. St Lucia	17	February 28, 1990.
20. St Vincent's and Grenadines	22	December 31, 1989.
21. Trinidad and Tobago	557	December 31, 1989.
22. Turks and Caicos Isles	8	December 31, 1988.

Asia

Recent data indicate that the total number of HIV infected persons in Asia has risen from virtually nil two years ago to an estimated current total of at least 500,000 (July 1990).

1. Afghanistan	No	cases by February 15, 1990.
2. Bangladesh	No	cases by November 30, 1989.
3. Burma	No	cases by November 30, 1989.
4. China	3	September 30, 1988.

5. Taiwan	14	September 30, 1989.
6. Hong Kong	22	February 28, 1990.
7. India	44	February 28, 1990.
8. Indonesia	7	February 28, 1990.
9. Japan	189	March 28, 1990. Estimated up to eleven thousand infected.
10. Kampuchea	No	cases by March 31, 1987.
11. North Korea	No	cases by September 30, 1989.
12. South Korea	5	October 8, 1989.
13. Laos	No	cases by March 31, 1987.
14. Macao	No	cases by January 18, 1990.
15. Malaysia	12	January 31, 1990. Some drug addicts infected.
16. Maldives	No	cases by September 30, 1989.
17. Mongolia	No	cases by March 2, 1990.
18. Nepal	2	January 16, 1990.
19. Pakistan	13	February 15, 1990.
20. Philippines	26	July 31, 1989. Many infected prostitutes near United States Navy Bases.
21. Singapore	15	January 31, 1988.
22. Sri Lanka	4	January 22, 1990.
23. Thailand	37	March 15, 1990. Now believed to have a severe and rapidly-growing problem. Estimated 50–100,000 infected drug users, up from only 1,000 two years ago. Many more suspected due to sexual tourism.
24. Vietnam	No	cases by September 8, 1988.

Table 1: Adult/adolescent AIDS cases by sex, exposure category, and race/ethnicity, reported up to April 1990, United States

Male exposure category	White, not Hispanic No. (%)	Black, not Hispanic No. (%)	Hispanic No. (%)	Asian/Pacific Islander No. (%)	American Indian/ Alaskan Native No. (%)	Total No. (%)
Male homosexual/bisexual contact	56,169 (80)	12,927 (44)	8,257 (47)	600 (81)	90 (62)	78,212 (66)
Intravenous (IV) drug use (heterosexual)	4,268 (6)	10,242 (35)	6,921 (39)	21 (3)	15 (10)	21,530 (18)
Male homosexual/bisexual contact and IV drug use	5,261 (8)	2,349 (8)	1,289 (7)	13 (2)	24 (16)	8,948 (8)
Haemophilia/coagulation disorder	957 (1)	74 (0)	87 (0)	15 (2)	6 (4)	1,143 (1)
Heterosexual contact:	420 (1)	2,030 (7)	217 (1)	6 (1)	1 (1)	2,678 (2)
Sex with IV drug user	*270*	*545*	*147*	*1*	*1*	*964*
Sex with person with haemophilia	*4*	*1*	–	–	–	*5*
Born in Pattern-II[6] country	*2*	*1,318*	*7*	*3*	–	*1,333*
Sex with person born in Pattern-II country	*24*	*24*	*4*	–	–	*52*
Sex with transfusion recipient with HIV infection	*19*	*9*	*1*	–	–	*30*
Sex with HIV-infected person, risk not specified	*101*	*133*	*58*	*2*	–	*294*
Receipt of blood transfusion, blood components, or tissue[7]	1,449 (2)	273 (1)	156 (1)	42 (6)	1 (1)	1,925 (2)
Other/undetermined[8]	1,411 (2)	1,282 (4)	824 (5)	44 (6)	9 (6)	3,580 (3)
Male subtotal	69,935(100)	29,167(100)	17,751(100)	741(100)	146(100)	118,016(100)

Table 2: Female exposure category

IV drug use	1,349 (41)	3,646 (57)	1,278 (52)	11 (17)	15 (56)	6,312 (52)
Haemophilia/coagulation disorder	23 (1)	4 (0)	1 (0)	–	–	28 (0)
Heterosexual contact:	919 (28)	2,006 (32)	889 (36)	25 (38)	7 (26)	3,854 (31)
Sex with IV drug user	*480*	*1,168*	*747*	*11*	*3*	*2,415*
Sex with bisexual male	*210*	*126*	*48*	*8*	*1*	*392*
Sex with person with haemophilia	*48*	*5*	*1*	*1*	–	*55*
Born in Pattern-II[b] country	*1*	*482*	*3*	*1*	–	*488*
Sex with person born in Pattern-II country	*3*	*34*	*1*	–	–	*38*
Sex with tranfusion recipient with HIV infection	*51*	*8*	*9*	*1*	–	*69*
Sex with HIV-infected person, risk not specified	*126*	*183*	*80*	*5*	*3*	*397*
Receipt of blood transfusion, blood components, or tissue	787 (24)	241 (4)	140 (6)	23 (35)	2 (7)	1,194 (10)
Other/undetermined	234 (7)	460 (7)	136 (6)	7 (11)	3 (11)	848 (7)
Female subtotal	3,312(100)	6,357(100)	2,444(100)	86(100)	27(100)	12,236(100)
Total	**73,247**	**35,514**	**20,195**	**807**	**173**	**130,252**

Table 3: AIDS cases in adolescents and adults under age 25 by exposure category, reported May 1988 to April 1989, May 1989 to April 1990, and cumulative totals to April 1990, United States

	13–19 years old			20–24 years old		
	May 1988–Apr. 1989	May 1989–Apr. 1990	Cumulative total	May 1988–Apr. 1989	May 1989–Apr. 1990	Cumulative total
Exposure category	No. (%)	No. (%)	No. (%)	No. (%)	No. (%)	No. (%)
Male homosexual/bisexual contact	32 (28)	33 (24)	145 (28)	819 (57)	802 (51)	3,254 (57)
Intravenous (IV) drug use (female and heterosexual male)	17 (15)	15 (11)	59 (12)	236 (18)	292 (19)	903 (16)
Male homosexual/bisexual contact and IV drug use	5 (4)	3 (2)	23 (4)	116 (8)	135 (9)	534 (9)
Haemophilia/coagulation disorder	34 (30)	39 (28)	157 (31)	41 (3)	37 (2)	148 (3)
Heterosexual contact:	13 (11)	25 (18)	62 (12)	137 (10)	175 (11)	603 (9)
Sex with IV drug user	*7*	*17*	*37*	*87*	*96*	*271*
Sex with bisexual male	–	*1*	*3*	*12*	*6*	*43*
Sex with person with heamophilia	–	*1*	*1*	*4*	*7*	*14*
Born in Pattern-II country	*3*	*2*	*13*	*12*	*26*	*100*
Sex with person born in Pattern-II country	–	–	–	–	*4*	*6*
Sex with tranfusion recipient with HIV infection	–	–	–	–	*3*	*4*
Sex with HIV-infected person, risk not specified	*3*	*4*	*8*	*22*	*33*	*65*
Receipt of blood transfusion, blood components, or tissue	14 (12)	3 (2)	38 (7)	25 (2)	13 (1)	86 (2)
Undetermined[12]	–	19 (14)	29 (6)	57 (4)	106 (7)	242 (4)
Total	115(100)	137(100)	513(100)	1,431(100)	1,560(100)	5,670(100)

APPENDIX E

A Directory of AIDS Organisations

This is an incomplete list; a fuller list in any country can be obtained by contacting some of the organisations below. Inclusion in this list is not necessarily a recommendation.

Europe

ACET (AIDS Care Education & Training)
PO Box 1323, London W5 5TF, UK. Tel: 081 840 7879 Fax: 081 840 2616
A Christian charity giving practical help with home care and grants, in addition to providing a schools education programme. Active overseas also.

British Medical Association
Tavistock Square, London W1, UK. Tel: 071 387 4499

Bureau of Hygiene and Tropical Diseases
Keppel Street, London WC1E 7HT, UK. Tel: 071 636 8636 Extension 275
Caroline Akehurst will advise on wide variety of very useful AIDS bulletins.

Body Positive
51b Philbeach Gardens, Earls Court, London SW5 9EB, UK. Tel: 071 835 1045
Provides many services including: drop-in centre, counselling, support groups, grants, and transport.

Christian Action on AIDS
PO Box 76, Hereford, HR1 1JX, UK. Tel: 0432 268167
This organisation aims to inform religious groups about AIDS.

Christian Medical Fellowship
157 Waterloo Road, London SE1 8XN, UK. Tel: 071 928 4694
Has a growing range of AIDS booklets.

Crusaid
21a Upper Tachbrook Street, London SW1V 1SN, UK. Tel: 071 834 7566
To raise and distribute funds for the support and care of people with AIDS/HIV.

Frontliners
52–54 Grays Inn Road, London WC1X 8JU, UK. Tel: 071 404 4324
A support group to provide information, advice, counselling and grants.

London Lighthouse
111–117 Lancaster Road, London W11 1QT, UK. Tel:071 792 1200
A major residential and support centre for people affected by AIDS which provides an integrated range of services.

Mildmay Mission Hospital
Hackney Road, London E2 7NA, UK. Tel: 071 739 2331
A Christian charity providing residential/palliative care, day care and home care.

National AIDS Trust
14th Floor, Euston Tower, 286 Euston Road, London NW1 3DN, UK. Tel: 071 388 1188 Extension 3200
Promotes and coordinates voluntary initiatives dealing with a wide range of issues.

Panos Institute
8 Alfred Place, London WC1E 7EB, UK. Tel: 071 631 1590
An AIDS and Devolopment Information Unit for developing countries.

SCODA (Standing Conference On Drug Abuse)
1–4 Matton Place, London C1N 8ND, UK. Tel: 071 430 2341
Coordinating body for non-statutory services; giving advice on referrals, training, funding, producing leaflets and conferences.

Scottish AIDS Monitor (SAM)
PO Box 48, Edinburgh EH1 3SA, UK. Tel: 031 557 3885
Provides information, education and support in all matters relating to HIV and AIDS.

Terrence Higgins Trust
52–54 Grays Inn Road, London, WC1X 8JU, UK. Tel: 071 831 0330
Offers counselling, support groups, helpline, legal advice, health education, and volunteer projects.

World Health Organisation (AIDS project)
Avenue Appia 1211, Geneva 27, Switzerland. Tel: 010 41 2291 21 11
Coordinates global HIV/AIDS prevention and control programmes.

United States

ACCT (AIDS Crisis and Christians Today)

PO Box 24647, Nashville, Tennessee 37202–4647; (615) 371 1616; Fax (615) 370 0764.

American Foundation for AIDS Research (AmFAR)

5900 Wilshire Blvd., 2nd Floor, East Satellite, Los Angeles, California 90036; 213/857–5900; and 40 West 57th Street, Suite 406, New York, New York 10019; 212/333–3118.

A private, not-for-profit organisation providing funding for research into the cure, prevention, and treatment of AIDS. It also produces educational materials.

Coming Home Hospice

c/o Visiting Nurses Association, Jeannie Martin, Director, 115 Diamond Street, Castro District, San Francisco, California 94102; 415/861–8705 or 415/285–5619.

Magnificent training manual for AIDS hospices and home care for $50 (excluding postage).

Mothers of AIDS Patients (MAP)

PO Box 3132, San Diego, California 92103; 619/293–3985 or 619/576–6366.

Started by three mothers who lost children to AIDS. It offers emotional support to families of people with AIDS, provides information about the disease, and assists people with AIDS who have been rejected or are isolated from their families.

National AIDS Network (NAN)

1012 14th Street NW, Suite 601, Washington, D.C. 20005; 202/347–0390.

The National AIDS Network consists of community-based AIDS organisations, hospitals, and educational facilities.

National Council of Churches/AIDS Task Force

475 Riverside Drive, Room 572, New York 10115; 212/870–2421.

Provides a resource and information packet for use by religious leaders in their congregations.

San Francisco AIDS Office

1111 Market Street, San Francisco, California 94103; 415/864–5571.

San Francisco General Hospital

Roberta Wilson, Oncology/AIDS Services, Ward 85, 995 Potrero Avenue, San Francisco, California 94110; 415/821–5531.

Publishes an excellent AIDS bulletin four times a year. No charge to have your name put on the mailing list.

Shanti Project
525 Howard Street, San Francisco, California 94105; 415/558–9644.
Has voluntary AIDS counselling, support, hostels, etc.

APPENDIX F

Further Reading

Suggested Popular Journals

See page 221 for list of scientific journals.

The best information by far is produced by the Bureau of Hygiene and Tropical Diseases (tel. 071 636 8636, ext. 275). Three publications:

(1) *AIDS Newsletter* 17 issues per year. Four regular sections: News and media—UK; News from abroad; Social and occupational; Science and medicine. Other features include publications, meetings and full indexing. It aims to provide health care professionals with an authoritative, accurate and up-to-date synopsis, in straightforward terms, of the latest developments in AIDS as reported by the lay, scientific and medical press.

(2) *Current AIDS Literature* (formerly *AIDS and Retroviruses Update* 1986–87) Monthly annotated and classified bibliography of recent books and reports on AIDS, related retrovirus infections and the agents that cause them. Each issue contains an overview—a look at last month's publications—and editorial commentaries of the main sections— epidemiology, clinical, medical microbiology and social. For health care professionals, public health workers and researchers.

(3) *WHO AIDS Technical Bulletin* contains extended précis of key papers with expert comment, abstracts of important articles and annotations of other relevant items, supplemented by statistics and other information as appropriate. French and Spanish editions to be published. For professionals working on AIDS in developing countries who do not have regular access to the original literature. Published by the Bureau of Hygiene and Tropical Diseases in collaboration with the World Health Organisation.

'AIDS Letter,' Royal Society of Medicine: Twenty-five issues a year of practical up-to-date information for people who have AIDS. (1 Wimpole Street, London W1M 8AE.) Strictly confidential mailing list.

Morbidity and Morality Weekly Report, vol. 35, no. 53 (1986): 119–120. A summary of United States sources of information.

National AIDS Information Clearinghouse, PO Box 6003, Rockville, MD 20850, USA, is a centralised source of information on AIDS.

Suggested Books

AIDS and the Third World (Panos Dossier, 8 Alfred Place, London WC1E 7EB).

AIDS and HTLV III medical briefing. Terrence Higgins Trust on AIDS (London WC1N 3XX).

Aitken, Jerry and Steve. *How Will I Tell My Mother?* Thomas Nelson: 1988.

Barber, Cryil. *Your Marriage Can Last A Lifetime*. Thomas Nelson: 1989.

Barclay, William. *Ethics in a Permissive Society*. Fontana.

Coates, Gerald. *What on Earth Is This Kingdom?* Kingsway Publications: 1983.

Double, Don. *For Best Results Follow the Maker's Instructions*. Marshall Pickering: 1984.

Facts about AIDS for Drug Users. Terrence Higgins Trust on AIDS (London WC1N 3XX).

Foster, Richard. *Celebration of Discipline*. Hodder and Stoughton: 1978.

Hanratty, Dr J. *Control of Distressing Symptoms*. St Joseph's Hospice, Mare Street, Hackney, London.

Hinton, J. *Dying*. Penguin: 1972.

Houghton, John. *A Touch of Love—A Straightforward Guide to Sexual Happiness*. Kingway Publications: 1986.

Knowles, Andrew. *Finding Faith*. Lion Publishing.

Kubler-Ross, Elizabeth. *On Death and Dying*. Macmillan: 1969.

La Haye, Tim and Beverly. *The Act of Marriage – The Beauty of Sexual Love*. Zondervan Publishing: 1976.

Livesey, Roy. *Understanding Alternative Medicine*. New Wine Press.

McCloughry, Roy and Carol Bebawi. *AIDS: A Christian Response*. Grove Books, Ltd.

Murray-Parkes, Colin. *Bereavement*. Penguin.

Ortiz, Juan Carlos. *Living with Jesus Today*. SPCK: 1982.

Pinching, Anthony, ed. 'AIDS and HIV Infection,' *Clinics in Immunology and Allergy*. W.B.Saunders, 1986. A good medical book on AIDS.

Watson, David. *Fear No Evil*. Hodder and Stoughton. A description of the author's own dying.

Wheat, Dr Ed. *Intended for Pleasure – Sex Technique and Sexual Fulfillment in Christian Marriage*. Scripture Union: 1977.

Wheat, Dr Ed. *Love Life*.

Wimber, John. *Power Healing*. Hodder and Stoughton.

APPENDIX G

An Awareness List of Scientific Journal Articles

Advisory Committee on Dangerous Pathogens (United Kingdom)

Revised guidelines (June 1986). *LAV/HTLV-III—the causative agent of AIDS and related conditions.*

AIDS

Marmor, M., Des Jarlais, D.C., Cohen, H., *et al.*, 1.1 (1987): 39–44. *Risk factors for infection with human immunodeficiency virus among intravenous drug abusers in New York City.*

Carswell, J.W., 1:4 (1987): 223–227. *HIV infection in healthy persons in Uganda.*

Lefrere, J.J., 1:4 (1987): 258–259. *HIV infection and Gc: absence of relationship (i.e. no genetic or racial susceptibility).*

Berkley, S. *et. al.*, 3:2 (1989): 79–85. *Surveillance for AIDS in Uganda.*

AIDS Bulletin (United Kingdom)

UK Institute of Actuaries, no. 3 (1988): 62. *Report from the Institute of Actuaries AIDS working party.*

Aidsfile

Volberding, P., 1:1 (1986). *Current status of antiviral therapy for AIDS.*

Leoung, G., 1:2. *Prophylactic therapy for* Pneumocystis carinii *pneumonia.*

Hollander, H., 1:3 (1986). *Neurological complications of AIDS.*

Varmus, H., 1:3 (1987). *Renaming the AIDS virus: clarity or confusion.*

Dilley, J., 2:1 (1987): 6–7. *Diagnosis and treatment of major depression in AIDS.*

Wofsy, C., 2:2 (1987): 1. *Advances in treatment of* Pneumocystis carinii *pneumonia.*

Grossman, M., 2:2 (1987): 3–4. *AIDS in children.*

AIDS-Forschung

Leenen, H.J.J., 1:9 (1986): 505–513. *Law and AIDS.*

Schkund, G.H., 1:10 (1986): 564–570. *Legal aspects of AIDS, part 2.*

Gonzalez, J., Koch, M., 1:11 (1986): 621–630. *The role of the transients for the prognostic analysis of AIDS and the anciennity distribution of AIDS*

patients.
2:1 (1987): 5–25. *AIDS in Africa.*
Herzberg, R.D., 2:2 (1987): 52–55. *AIDS as a punishable offense.*
Frosner, G.G., 2:2 (1987): 61–65. *What can be done against further spread of AIDS?*
Chermann, J.C., Barre-Sinoussi, F., Henin, Y., Marechal, V., 2:2 (1987): 85–86. *HIV inactivation by a spermicide containing benzalkonium chloride.*
Jurisdiction Regional Munich Court, 2:11 (1987): 648–651.
Velimirovic, B., 3:7 (1988): 392–401. *Exploitation of AIDS patients: trading with false hopes, quackery, drugs, and unauthorised therapies.*

AIDS Newsletter
2:11 (1987). *Report on church and homosexuality.*

AIDS Research
Buimovici-Klein, E., Ong, K.R., Lange, M., *et al.*, 2:4 (1986): 279–283. *Reverse transcriptase activity (RTA) in lymphocyte cultures of AIDS patients treated with HPA-23.*

AIDS Weekly Surveillance Report (United States)
29 June 1987.

Alternatives to Laboratory Animals (ATLA)
Editorial, 15:3 (1988): 176–179. *Salvation or extinction of the chimpanzee: the final struggle begins.*

American Journal of Epidemiology
Chmiel, J.S., *et al.*, 126:4 (1987): 568–577. *Factors associated with prevalent HIV infection in the multicentre AIDS cohort study.*

American Journal of Medicine
Goldman, R., Lang, W., Lyman, D., 81:6 (1986): 1122–1123. *Acute AIDS viral infection.*
Teich, S.A., Tay, S., Friedman, A./H., Schmitterer, M.E., 82:1 (1987): 151–152. *Viral particles in the conjunctiva of a patient with the acquired immune deficiency syndrome.*
Pekovic, D., Ajdukovic, D., Tsoukas, C., Lapointe, N., Michaud, J., Gilmore, N., Gornitsky, M., 82:1 (1987): 188–189. *Detection of human immunosuppressive [sic] virus in salivary lymphocytes from dental patients with AIDS.*

American Journal of Preventive Medicine
Dull, H.B., 4:4 (1988): 239–240. *Behind the AIDS mailer.*

American Journal of Public Health
76 (1986): 1325–1330. [Report on the rapid spread of the disease in the United States.]
Martin, J.L., 77:5 (1987): 578–581. *The impact of AIDS on gay male*

sexual behaviour patterns in New York City.
Drotman, D.P., 77:2 (1987): 143. *Now is the time to prevent AIDS.*
Kegelles, *et al.*, 78:4 (1988): 460–461. *Sexually active adolescents and condoms: changes over one year in knowledge, attitudes and use.*
McCusker, *et al.*, 78:4 (1988): 462–467. *Effects of HIV antibody test knowledge on subsequent sexual behaviours in a cohort of homosexually active men.*

American Review of Respiratory Diseases
Bibgy, T., *et al.*, 133 (1986): 515–518. *Usefulness of induced sputum in the diagnosis of* Pneumocystis carinii *pneumonia in patients with AIDS.*

Annales de L'Institut Pasteur
Merlin, M., *et al.*, 138:4 (1987): 503–510. *Epidemiology of HIV infection among ... Central African populations.*

Annales de la Société Belge de Médecine Tropicale
Mann, J.M., Francis, H., Quinn, T.C., *et al.*, 66:3 (1986): 345–350. *HIV seroincidence in a hospital worker population: Kinshasa, Zaire.*

Annals of Internal Medicine
Burke, D.S., Redfield, R.S., 105:6 (1986): 968. *Classification of infections with human immunodeficiency virus.*
Marmor, M., Weiss, L.R., Lyden, M., *et al.*, 105:6 (1986): 969. *Possible female-to-female transmission of human immunodeficiency virus.*
Kumar, P., Pearson, J.E., Martin, D.H., *et al.*, 106:2 (1987): 244–245. *Transmission of human immunodeficiency virus by transplantation of a renal allograft with development of the acquired immunodeficiency syndrome.*

Antiviral Research
De Clerq, E., 7:1 (1987): 1–10. *Suramin in the treatment of AIDS: mechanism of action.*

Archives of Dermatology
El-Akkad, S., Bull, C.A., El-Senoussi, M.A., Griffin, J.T., Amer, M., 122:22 (1986): 1396–1399. *Kaposi's sarcoma and its management by radiotherapy.*

Archives of Internal Medicine
Dwyer, J.M., Wood, C.C., McNamara, J., Kinder, B, 147:3 (1987): 513–517. *Transplantation of thymic tissue into patients with AIDS: an attempt to reconstitute the immune system.*

British Dental Journal
Kay, E.J., 162:2 (1987): 53. *Acceptance of hepatitus B vaccine by GDP's in the United Kingdom.*
Walsh, J.P., 162:10 (1987): 375. *AIDS and the dentist.*

British Journal of Psychiatry

Jacob, K.S., John, J.K., Verghese, A., John, T.J., 150 (1987): 412–413. *AIDS-phobia.*

Segal, M., 152 (MOW) (1988): 244. *AIDS update.*

British Medical Journal

(1984): 1. *ABC of Sexually Transmitted Diseases.* (Book of reprinted articles.)

Mortimer, P.P., Jesson, W.J., *et al.*, 290 (1985): 1176–1178. *Prevalence of antibody to human T lymphotropic virus type III by risk group and area, United Kingdom 1978–84.*

Johnson, A., Adler, M., Crown, J., 293 (1986): 489–492. *The acquired immune deficiency syndrome and epidemic of infection with human immunodeficiency virus: costs of care and prevention in an inner London district.*

Porter, R., 293 (1986): 1589–1590. *History says no to the policeman's response to AIDS.*

Smith, T., 294 (1987): 6. *AIDS: a doctor's duty.*

Walker, M.M., Griffiths, C.E.M., Weber, J., *et al.*, 294 (1987): 29–32. *Dermatological conditions in HIV infection.*

Kay, L.A., 294 (1987): 137–139. *The need for autologous blood transfusion.*

Denning, D.W., Anderson, J., Rudge, P., Smith, H., 294 (1987): 143–144. *Acute myelopathy associated with primary infection with human immunodeficiency virus.*

Doll, R., 294 (1987): 244. *A proposal for doing prevalence studies of AIDS.*

Cooke, M.W., 294 (1987): 246. *AIDS: a doctor's duty.*

Slater, N.G.P., 294 (1987): 307. *Safeguarding the blood supply.*

Moss, A.R., 294 (1987): 389–390. *AIDS and intravenous drug use: the real heterosexual epidemic.*

Walker, E., 294 (1987): 433. *Testing wind-instrument reeds: What risk is there of infection being transmitted by this practice?*

Guy, P.J., 294 (1987): 445. *Is testing for HIV without consent ever warranted?*

Smelt, G.J.C., 294 (1987): 446. *The possibility of AIDS.*

Robertson, J.R., Skidmore, C., 294 (1987): 571. *AIDS and intravenous drug use.*

Wood, P.J.W., 294 (1987): 571–572. *AIDS and intravenous drug use.*

Crawford, R.J., Mitchell, R., Burnett, A.K., Follett, E.A.C., 294 (1987): 572. *Who may give blood?*

294 (1987): 647. *AIDS a doctor's duty.*

Hill, M., Mayon-White, D., 294 (1987): 649. *AIDS publicity.*

West, N., 294 (1987): 772. *Identity cards for patients infected with HIV?*

Carne, C.A., Weller, I.V.D., Loveday, C., Adler, M.W., 294 (1987):

868–869. *From persistent generalised lymphadenopathy to AIDS: who will progress?*
Goldberg, D.J., 294 (1987): 906. *AIDS and intravenous drug use.*
Smith, J.W.G., 294 (1987): 1033. *HIV transmitted by kissing.*
Fitzgerald, M.R., 294 (1987): 1160. *Testing for HIV without permission.*
Pinching, A.J., 294 (1987): *AIDS and the heterosexual epidemic.*
Comfort, A., 294 (1987): 1356. *Preventing AIDS.*
294 (1987): 1595–1597. *Prospective study of clinical, laboratory and ancillary staff with accidental exposures to blood or body fluids from patients infected with HIV.*
Editorial, 295 (1987): 284–285. *Burnout.*
Brettle, *et al.*, 295 (1987): L421. *Human immunodeficiency virus an drug misuse: the Edinburgh experience.*
Editorial, 295 (1987): 454. *Gender reassignment today.*
296 (1988): 244. *Aids update.*
Moss, *et al.*, 296 (12 March 1988): 745–750. *Seropositivity and the development of AIDS or ARC. Three year follow-up of the San Francisco Hospital cohort.*
Johnson, A., 296 (1988): 1017–1020. *Heterosexual transmission of HIV.*
McCormick, A., 296 (1988): 1289–1292. *Trends in mortality statistics in England and Wales with particular reference to AIDS from 1984 to 1987.*
Dudley, H.A., Sim, A., 296 (1988): 1449–1450. *AIDS: a bill of rights for the surgical team?*
297 (1988): 859. *HIV infection in Scotland.*
McMillan, A., 297 (1988): 873–874. *Editorial: HIV in prisons—action, research, and condoms needed.*
Loveday, C. *et al.*, 298 (1989): 419–422. *HIV in patients attending an STD clinic in London, 1982–1987.*
Wright, J.D.; Pearl, L., 300 (1990); 99–103 *Young People and drug abuse.*

Bulletin of the World Health Association
Nguyen-Dinh, P., *et al.*, 65:5 (1987): 607–613. *Absence of association between ... malaria and HIV infection in children in ... Zaire.*

Canadian Medical Association Journal
Quaggin, A., 136:2 (1987): 192–193. *Get prepared for more cases of AIDS during pregnancy.*
Trent, B., 136:2 (1987): 194. *AIDS has created a new form of bereavement.*
Rogan, E., *et al.*, 137:7 (1987): 637–638. *A case of AIDS before 1980 in Zaire.*
Cohen, L., 137:10 (1987): 932–933. *Cashing in on AIDS: turning a disaster into a business proposition.*
Frank, J.W., *et al.*, 138:4 (1988): 287–288. *Testing for HIV infection: ethical considerations revisted.*
Noel, G.E., 138:6 (1988): 490. *Transmission of HIV: surgical clips to close wounds.*

Cancer Research

Duesberg, Peter H., 47 (1 March 1987): 1199:1220. *Retroviruses as carcinogens and pathogens: expectations and reality.*

Cell

Maddon, P.J., Dalgleish, A.G., McDouglas, J.S., Clapham, P.R., Weiss, R.A., Axel, R., 47:3 (1986): 333–348. *The T4 gene encodes the AIDS virus receptor and is expressed in the immune system and the brain.*

Chest

Caughey, *et al.*, 88 (1985): 658–662. *Nonbronchoscopic broncho-alveolar lavage for the diagnosis of* Pneumocystis carinii *pneumonia in AIDS.*

Clinical Microbiology Newsletter

9:2 (1987): 15. *Regarding the discontinuation of labelling clinical specimens as 'hazardous'.*

Clinics in Immunology and Allergy

Pinching, A.J. (guest editor), 6:3 (1986): 441–687. *AIDS and HIV infection.*

Deutsche Medizinische Wochenschrift

Deinhardt, F., 111:40 (1986): 1540. *Outcome of LAV/HTLV-III infection.*

European Journal of Clinical Microbiology

Clumeck, N., 5:6 (1986): 609–611. *Heterosexual transmission of AIDS: no time for complacency.*

Genitourinary Medicine

Donovan, B., Tindall, B., Cooper, D., 62:6 (1986): 390–392. *Brachiopractic eroticism and tranmission of retrovirus associated with acquired immune deficiency syndrome (AIDS).*

Health and Safety Journal

Ingeldew, D., Holbourn, A., (1987): 33. *AIDS risk for NHS staff greater outside work.*

Holistic Medicine

Kermani, K.S., 2:4 (1987): 203–215. *Stress, emotions, autogenic training and AIDS: a holistic approach to the management of HIV-infected individuals.*

Immunobiology

Oettgen, H.F., Real, F.X., Krown, S.E., 172:3/5 (1986): 269–274. *Treatment of AIDS-ssociated Kaposi's sarcoma with recombinant alpha interferon.*

Gramatzki, M., Nusslein, H., Burmester, G.R., *et al.*, 172:3/5 (1986): 438–447. *Intralymphatic interlenkin 2 treatment in patients with acquired immunodeficiency syndrome: preliminary experience in three cases.*

Immunology Today

Brandtzael, P., 8:1 (1987): 8–9, *HIV is an inappropriate name for the AIDS virus.*

International Journal of Cancer

Miller, G.J., Pegram, S.M., Kirkwood, B.R., *et al.*, 38:6 (1986): 801–808. *Ethnic composition, age and sex, together with location and standard of housing as determinants of HTLV-I infection in an urban Trinidadian community.*

Journal of Infection

Gill, O.N., 16:1 (1988): 3–23. *The hazard of infection from the shared communion cup—shows no evidence of any disease transmitted, let alone HIV.*

Journal of Infectious Diseases

Martin, L., *et al.*, 152:2 (1985): 400–403. *Disinfection and anactivation of the human T lymphotropic virus type III/lymphadenopathy-associated virus.*

Douglas, J.M.Jr., Rogers, M., Judson, F.N., 154:2 (1986): 331–334. *The effect of asymptomatic infection with HTLV-III on the response of anogenital warts to intralesional treatment with recombinant and interferon.*

Taylor, J.M.G., Schwartz, K., Detels, R., 154:4 (1986): 694–697. *The time from infection with human immunodeficiency virus (HIV) to the onset of AIDS.*

Laskin, O.L., Stahl-Bayliss, C.M., Kalman, C.M., Rosecan, L.R., 155:2 (1987): 323–326. *Use of ganciclovir to treat serious cytomegalovirus infections in patients with AIDS.*

Napoli, V.M., McGowan, J.E.Jr., 155:4 (1987): 828. *How much blood is in a needlestick?*

Bacchetti, P., Osmond, D., *et al.*, 157:5 (1988): 1044–1047. *Survival patterns of the first five hundred patients with AIDS in San Francisco.*

Journal of Occupational Medicine

Lewy, R., 30:7 (1988): 578–579. *AIDS in the workplace: guidelines.*

Journal of Pediatrics

Jaffee, L., *et al.*, 112:6 (1988): 1005–1007. *Anal intercourse and knowledge of AIDS among minority-group female adolescents.*

Journal of Social Issues

Freudenberger, 30 (1984): 159–165. *Staff burnout.*

Journal of the American Medical Association

Resnic, *et al.*, 255 (1986): 1887–1891. *Stability and inactivation of HTLV-III/LAV under clinical and laboratory conditions.*

USA, American Medical Association, Council on Scientific Affairs, 256:17 (1986): 2378–2380. *Autologous blood transfusions.*

Guarner, J., Del Rio, C., Slade, B., 256:22 (1986): 3092. *Tuberculosis as a manifestation of the acquired immunodeficiency syndrome.*
Leiderman, I.Z., 256:22 (1986): 3092. *A child with HIV infection.*
Winkelstein, W., Lyman, D.M., Padian, N., *et al.*, 257:3 (1987): 321–325. *Sexual practices and risk of infection by the human immunodeficiency virus: the San Francisco's Men's Health Study.*
Fischl, M.A., *et al.*, 257 (1987): 640–644. *Evaluation of heterosexual partners, children, and household contacts of adults with AIDS.*
Schmidt, P.J., 257:7 (1987): 928–929. *Autologous blood transfusion.*
Haugen, R.K., Hill, G.E., 257:9 (1987): 1211–1214. *A large-scale autologous blood programme in a community hospital: contribution to the community's blood supply.*
Michailis, B.A., 257:10 (1987): 1327. *Recovery of human immunodeficiency virus from serum.*
Potterat, J.J., Phillips, L., Muth, J.B., 257:13 (1987): 1727. *Lying to military physicians about risk factors for HIV infections.*
Greenberg, A., *et al.*, 259:4 (1988): 545–549. *Association between malaria, blood tranfusions, and HIV seropositivity in a pediatric population in Kinshasa, Zaire.*
Marzuk, P.M., *et al.*, 259:9 (1988): 1333–1337. *Increased risk of suicide in persons with AIDS.*
259:9 294 (1989): 1360–1361. *Ethical issues involved in the growing AIDS crisis – American Medical Association Council on Ethical and Judicial Affairs.*
Rutherford, G.W. *et al.*, 259:15 (1988): 2235. *Impact of the revised AIDS case definition on AIDS reporting in San Francisco.*
Levy, J., 259:20 (1988): 3037–3038. *Transmission of AIDS: the case of the infected cell.*
Hegarty, J.D., *et al.*, (1988): 1901–1905. *Medical care costs of HIV-infected Harlem children.*
Selwyn, P.A. *et al.*, 261:9 (1989): 1289–1294. *Prospective study of HIV and pregnancy in IVDUS.*
Lemp, G.R., *et al.*, 263:3 (1990): 402–406. *Survival trends for patients with AIDS.*

Journal of the Medical Defence Union
Cooke, E.M., Tomkins, C.M., 2:3 (1986): 21–22. *AIDS: more medico-legal problems.*

Journal of the Royal Society of Medicine
Editorial, 80 (1987): 265. *Our response to AIDS.*
Boyd, K., 80 (1987): 281–383. *The moral challenge of AIDS.*

Lancet
Dubois, R.M., Braithwaite, M.A., Mikhail, J.R., *et al.*, 2 (1981): 1339. Primary *Pneumocystis carinii* and cytomegalovirus infections.

Bygberg, I.C., 1 (1983): 925. *AIDS in a Danish surgeon.*
Marmor, Friedman-Kien, Laubenstein, *et al.*, 1 (1983): 1083–1087. *Risk factors for Kaposi's sarcoma in homosexual men.*
Spire, B., *et al.*, 2 (1984): 899–901. *Inactivation of lymphadenopathy-associated virus by chemical disinfectants.*
Spire, B., *et al.*, 2 (1985): 188–189 *Inactivation of lymphadenopathy-associated virus by heat, gamma rays, and ultraviolet light.*
Carne, C., Weller, I., Sutherland, S., *et al.*, 1 (1985): 1261–1262. *Rising prevalence of human T-lymphotropic virus type III (HTLV-III) infection in homosexual men in London.*
Wofsy, C., *et al.*, 1 (1986): 527–528. *Isolation of AIDS-associated retrovirus from genital secretions of women with anitbodies to the virus.*
Koenig, R.E., Gantier, T., Levy, J.A., 2 (1986): 694. *Horizontal transmission of HIV infection between two siblings.*
Neisson-Vermont, C., *et al.*, 2 (1986): 814. *Needlestick HIV seroconversion in a nurse.*
Editorial, 2 (1986): 1430–1431. *An unexpected new virus.*
Wetterberg, L., Alexius, B., Saaf, J., Sonnerborg, A., Britton, S., Pert, C., 1 (1987): 159. *Peptide T in treatment of AIDS.*
Brucker, G., Brun-Vezinet, F., Rosenheim, M., Rey, M.A., Katlama, C., Gentilini, M., 1 (1987): 223. *HIV-2 infection in two homosexual men in France.*
Mortimer, P.P., 1 (1987): 280–281. *Viral cause of Kaposi's sarcoma?*
Kelly, J.A., St. Lawrence, J.S., 1 (1987): 323. *Caution about condoms in prevention of AIDS.*
Tovey, S.J., 1 (1987): 567. *Condoms and AIDS prevention.*
Kelly, D.A., Hallett, R.J., Saeed, A., Levinsky, R.J., Strobel, S., 1 (1987): 806–807. *Prolonged survival and late presentation of vertically transmitted HIV infection in childhood.*
Mitchell, W.M., Montefiori, D.C., Robinson, W.E.Jr., Strayer, D.R., Carter, W.A., 1 (1987): 890–892. *Mismatched double-stranded RNA (ampligen) reduces concentration of zidovudine (azidothymidine) required for* invitro *inhibition of human immunodeficiency virus.*
Cook, C.C.H., 1 (1987): 920–921. *Syringe exchange.*
Marshall, G.S., Barbour, S.D., Plotkin, S.A., 1 (1987): 446–447. *AIDS in a child without antibody to HIV.*
Lawrence, A.G., Singaratnam, A.E., 1 (1987): 982–983. *Changes in sexual behavior and incidence of gonorrhea.*
Clarke, J.A., 1 (1987): 983. *HIV transmission and skin grafts.* 1 (1987): 999–1002. *Genetics and AIDS?*
Lucas, A., 1 (1987): 1092–1093. *AIDS and human milk bank closures.*
Srinivasan, A., York, D., Bohan, C., 1 (1987): 1094–1095. *Lack of HIV replication in arthropod cells.*
McKeganey, Bloor, 1 (1987): 1323. *Needle exchange* 1 (1987): 1448–1449. *African fertility rites and AIDS.*

Monzon, O., Capellan, J., 2 (1987): 40–41. *Female-to-female tranmission of HIV.*
2 (1987): 166. *T4 cells in skin.*
Konotey-Ahulu, F., 2 (1987): 206. *Point of view: AIDS in Africa, misinformation and disinformation.*
Paloczi, 1 (2/4 January 1988): 65. *HIV transmission from female to male at improperly protected sexual intercourse.*
Stehr, Green, *et al.*, 1 (March 1988): 520–521. *Potential effect of revising the CDC surveillance case definition for AIDS.*
Eales, L.J., Nye, K.E., Pinching, A.J., 1 (23 April 1988): 936. *Group specific compound and AIDS: erroneous data (i.e. no genetic or racial differences after all).*
Beral, V. *et al.*, (20 January 1990): 123 *Kaposi's sarcoma and AIDS (update).*
Smith *et al.*, (10 February 1990): 359: *Safe sex and contraception—a dilemma.*

Microbiology and Immunology
Ishida, T., Yamamoto, K., Shotake, T., Nozawa, K., Hayami, M., Hinuma, Y., 30:4 (1986): 315–321. *A field study of infection with human T-cell leukemia virus among African primates.*

Morbidity and Mortality Weekly Reports (United States)
30 (1981): 305–309.
35 (1988): 76–79.
35:45 (1986): 699–703. *Tuberculosis: United States, 1985.*
36:9 (1987): 133–135. *Tuberculosis and AIDS: Connecticut.*
6:12 (1987): 187–189. *Self-reported changes in sexual behaviors among homosexual and bisexual men from the San Francisco City Clinic cohort.*
39 (1990): 2: 20–22. *Years of potential life lost before age 65 and 85—US 1987 and 1988.*

Nature (United Kingdom)
Newmark, P., 324:304 (1986): *Problems with AIDS vaccines.*
Newmark, P. 324 (1986): 611. *AIDS in an African context.*
Ellrodt, A., Le Bras, P., 325 (1987): 765. *The hidden dangers of AIDS vaccination.*
Rees, M., 326 (1987): 343–345. *The sombre view of AIDS.*
326 (1987): 424. *Peptide T.*
Palc, J., 326 (1987): 533. *Settlement on AIDS finally reached between United States and Pasteur.*
Fox, C.H., 326 (1987): 636. *AIDS caused by a slow virus.*
Johnston, K., 327 (1987): 95. *WHO derides vaccine scare.*
Bloom, B.R., 327 (1987): 193. *AIDS vaccine strategies.*
Furth, P.A., 327 (1987): 193. *Heterosexual transmission of AIDS by male drug users.*

Ezzell, C., 327 (1987): 261. *Hospital workers have AIDS virus.*

Fuchs, D., *et al.*, 330 (1987): 702–703. *HIV vaccination and blood transfusion.*

Weiss, R., 331 (1988): 15. *Receptor molecule blocks HIV.*

Hussey, R., *et al.*, 331 (1988): 78–81. *A soluble CD4 protein selectively inhibits HIV replication and syncytium formation.*

Fisher, R.A., *et al.*, 331 (1988): 76–78. *HIV infection is blocked in intro by recombinent soluble CD4.*

Traunecker, A., 331 (1988): 84–86. *Soluble CD4 molecules neutralise HIV1.*

Saag, M.S., *et al.*, 334 (1988): 440–444. *Extensive variation of HIV type 1—invitro.*

Editorial, 334 (1988): 457. *More missed chances: President Ronald Reagan leaves tough decisions on AIDS to his successors.*

Edman, J.C., *et al.*, 334 (1988): 519–522. *Ribosomal RNA sequences show* Pneumocystis carinii *to be a member of the fungi.*

Nederlands Tijdschrift voor Geneeskunde

Van Griensven, G.J.P., Tielman, R.A.P., Goudsmit, J., Van der Noordaa, J., De Wolf, F., Coutinho, R.A., 130:48 (1986): 2178–2189. *LAV/HTLV-III infection among homosexual males in the Netherlands: prevalence and psychosocial factors.*

New England Journal of Medicine

McCray, E., 314 (1986): 1127–1132. *The cooperative needlestick surveillance group. Occupational risk of AIDS among health care workers.*

Surgenor, D. MacN., 316:9 (1987): 543–544. *The patient's blood is the safest blood.*

Osterholm, M.T., MacDonald, K.L., Danila, R.N., Hentry, K., 316:16 (1987): 1024. *Sexually transmitted disease in victims of sexual assault.*

Jagger, J., *et al.*, 319:5 (1988): 284–288.

Mann, J.M., Chin, J., 319:5 (1988): 302–303. *AIDS: a global perspective.*

Wempen, P.M., 319:5 (1988): 308. *Equipment modifications to reduce needle sticks.*

Weiss, R., Thier, S.O., 319:5 (1988): 1010–1012. *HIV testing is the answer—what's the question?*

Schneiderman, L.J., Spragg, R.G., 318:15 (1988): 984–988. *Ethical considerations in discontinuing mechanical ventilation (one patient with AIDS).*

Back, M.C., 320:9 (1989): 594–595. *Failure of zidovudine to maintain remission in patients with AIDS.*

Fahey *et al.*, 322 (3) 1990: 166–172: *Prognostic value of cellular and seriological markers in HIV.*

New Scientist

Kingman, S., 113 (26 March 1987): 38–39. *How you can catch it—and how you can't.*

Ferry, G., 113 (26 March 1987): 40–43. *AIDS in Africa.*

Koch, M., 113 (26 March 1987): 46–51. *The anatomy of the virus.*

(7 January 1988): 36–37. *Control campaign in Kenya kicks off with $3 million.*

(7 January 1988): 36–37. *'Safe sex' stops the spread of AIDS.*

Kingman, S., 117 (14 January 1988): 34–35. *How Africa must live with AIDS.*

Duesberg, P., 118 (28 April 1988): 34–35. *AIDS and the 'innocent' virus.*

Weber, J., 119 (5 May 1988): 32–33. *AIDS and the 'innocent' virus – a reply.*

Campbell, D. (12 November 1988): 26. *AIDS: patient power puts research on trial.*

Occupational Health Review

6:12 (1987). *AIDS and first aid.*

Parasitology Today

Piot, P., Schofield, C.J., 2;11 (1986): 294–295. *No evidence for arthropod transmission of AIDS.*

Pediatrics

Epstein, L.G., Sharer, L.R., Oleske, J.M., *et al.*, 78:4 (1986): 678–687. *Neurologic manifestations of human immunodeficiency virus infection in children.*

Gershon, A.A., 78:4, supplement II (1986): 764. *Live attenuated varicella vaccine use in immunocompromised children and adults. What happens to AIDS patients when they get chickenpox?*

Alexander-Rodriguez, T., Vermund, S.M., 80:4 (1987): 501–504. *Gonorrhea and syphilis in incarcerated urban adolescents: prevalence and physical signs.*

Pahwa, S., 7:5 (1988): 561–571. *HIV infection in children (review).*

American Academy of Pediatrics Committee on School Health in the United States, 82:2 (1988): 278–280.

Postgradute Doctor—Africa

Miller, D., 8:11 (1986): 336–344. *How to counsel patients about HIV disease: those who have it and those who fear it.*

PHLS Microbiology Digest

Greenaway, P.J., Farrar, G.H., 4:2 (1987): 26–30. *Prospects for an AIDS vaccine.*

Proceedings of the National Academy of Sciences of the U.S.A., 85:23 (1988): 9234–9237. *Effects of neutralising antibodies on ARC and AIDS.*

Quarterly Journal of Medicine

Jacobson, M.A., *et al.*, 67:254 (1988): 473–486. *Retinal and gastro-intestinal disease due to cytomegalovirus in patients with AIDS. Prevalence, natural history, and response to ganeiclovir therapy.*

Reviews of Infectious Diseases

Vogt, M., Hirsch, M.S., 8:6 (1986): 991–1000. *Prospects for an AIDS vaccine.*

Huminer, *et al.*, 9:6 (1987): 1102–1108. *AIDS in the pre-AIDS era.*

De Gruttola, V., Mayewr, K.H., 10:1 (1988): 138–150. *Assessing and modeling heterosexual spread of HIV in the United States.*

Des Jarlais, *et al.*, 10:1 (1988): 151–158. *HIV infection and IV drug abuse: critical issues in transmission dynamics, infection outcomes, and prevention.*

Scandinavian Journal of Infectious Diseases

Sonnet, J., *et al.*, 19:5 (1987): 511–517. *Early AIDS cases (Zaire and Burundi) 1962–1976.*

Gotzsche, P.C., Hording, M., 20:2 (1988): 233–234. *Condoms to prevent HIV transmission do not imply truly safe sex.*

Science (United States)

Barnes, D.M., 233 (1986): 1035. *Will an AIDS vaccine bankrupt the company that makes it?*

Koenig, S., Gendelman, H.E., Orenstein, J.M., *et al.*, 233 (1986): 1089–1093. *Detection of AIDS virus in macrophages in brain tissue from AIDS patients with encephalopathy.*

Barnes, D.M., 233 (1986): 1149–1153. *Strategies for an AIDS vaccine.*

Barnes, D.M., 235 (1987): 964. *AIDS stresses health care in San Francisco.*

Kolata, G., 235 (1987): 1138–1139. *Clinical trials planned for new AIDS drug.*

Vogt, M.W., Hartshorn, K.L., Furman, P.A., *et al.*, 235 (1987): 1376–1379. *Ribavirin antagonizes the effort of azidothymidine on HIV replication.*

Kolata, G., 235 (1987): 1462–1463. *Imminent marketing of AZT raises problems.*

Kolata, G., 236 (1987): 382. *How to ask about sex and get honest answers.*

Bloom, D.E., Carliner, G., 239 (5 February 1988) 604–610. *Economic impact of AIDS in the United States.*

Scientific American

Gallo, R.C., 255:6 (1986): 78–88. *The first human retrovirus.*

Gallo, R.C., 256:1 (1987): 38–48. *The AIDS virus.*

Wright, K., 258:2 (1988): 18–19. *Flying blind: testing an AIDS vaccine may be harder than inventing one.*

(October 1988). *Whole issue devoted to AIDS.*

Sexually Transmitted Disease

Haverkos, *et al.*, 12 (1985): 203–208. *Disease manifestation among homosexual men with AIDS: a possible role of nitrites in Kaposi's sarcoma.*

Tubercle

Duncanson, F.P., Hewlett, D. Jr., Maayan, S., *et al.*, 67:4 (1986): 295–302. *Mycobacterium tuberculosis infection in the acquired immunodeficiency syndrome: a review of fourteen patients.*

USA Public Health Reports

102 (1986): 341.

Vaccine

5:2 (1987): 155. *New nucleic acid encoding AIDS associated retrovirus polypeptide useful for vaccine preparation or for AIDS diagnosis.*

World Health Forum

Konde-Lule, J.K., 9:3 (1988): 384. *Group health education against AIDS in rural Uganda.*

APPENDIX H

Glossary of Terms

(Abbreviations are listed first: other terms follow)

AID: Artificial Insemination by Donor. Technique used to inject a man's semen into the womb of a woman. Used where the man is infertile (someone else donates sperm). A single donation of sperm has resulted in infection for the woman with HIV. The risks are quite high using conventional methods. Many gay men fancy the idea of being fathers even though they cannot bring themselves to have sex with a woman. They masturbate to produce semen which is then given to a semen bank. This anonymous bank is then used to provide semen for women wanting babies. Semen banks are now insisting on testing all donors for AIDS three months after the semen was donated. The semen can be stored almost indefinitely in liquid nitrogen.

AIDS: Acquired Immune Deficiency Syndrome.

ARC: AIDS Related Conditions (pre-AIDS syndrome), or AIDS Related Complex.

ARV: AIDS associated retrovirus (old name for HIV).

AZT: Antiviral drug currently being evaluated. Otherwise known as Zidovudine. Most effective drug discovered so far.

CD4: New experimental therapy injecting fragments similar to T4 white cell wall in order to mop up free virus in the blood.

CMV: See also Cytomegalovirus. Common cause of diarrhoea in AIDS.

CSF: See Cerebrospinal fluid.

DMFO: See Dimethylfluorornithine.

DNA: Deoxyribonucleic acid: complex making up genetic code (genes) contained in cell nucleus (brain).

ELISA: Enzyme Linked Immunosorbent Assay—a test used on blood or plasma before transfusion to detect infection with HIV.

GP: General Practitioner.

HCW: Health Care Workers.

HIV: Human Immunodeficiency Virus—new name for the

virus causing AIDS agreed to by an international scientific committee.

HPA-23: Anti-viral drug with slight effect on HIV but serious side-effects.

HTLV-III: Human T-Lymphotropic Virus type III (old name for HIV).

ICU: Intensive Care Unit.

Ig: Immunoglobulin or antibody.

ITU: Intensive Care Unit.

IV: Intravenous—drugs directly injected into a vein. Same as 'mainlining' or 'shooting' for drug abuse.

KS: Kaposi's sarcoma.

LAV: Lymphadenopathy Associated Virus (old name for HIV).

LSD: Drug causing hallucinations. Used to be popular in the sixties. People take it for an exaggerated perception of situations, sound, colour, and memories. It causes death due to the person's being unaware of risks and having unreal ideas, e.g., that they can fly so they jump out of a window. It may cause repeat 'trips' which can occur at any time without any warning some months after the initial experience. The drug has disappeared long ago from the body but it has damaged the brain in some bizarre way. A cousin of mine was given the drug by a doctor as part of a treatment for depression in the sixties. It has long been rejected for this and any other medical purpose. My cousin had a 'bad trip' which was extremely frightening. He had flashbacks at intervals for years.

NIR: No Identified Risk, i.e., not drug addict, homosexual, bisexual, no blood transfusions, etc. Often misapplied term—it is just that the person is too embarrassed to admit the truth.

NY: New York.

OD: Slang for overdose by drug users.

PCP: *Pneumocystis Carinii* Pneumonia.

PGL: Persistent Generalised Lymphadenopathy—large lymph nodes for several months. Early sign of infection.

RNA: Ribonucleic acid: carbon copy of DNA which is used to carry instructions from DNA throughout the cell. Retroviruses contain RNA.

STD: Sexually Transmitted Disease—same as VD.

TMP-SMX: Antibiotic used to treat pneumocystis chest infections. May affect bone marrow.

VD: Venereal Disease—same as STD.

Acyclovir:	Antiviral drug currently being evaluated.
Alpha-interferon:	Substance usually produced by T4 white cells. Being evaluated as an anti-AIDS drug.
Amphetamines:	Drugs which stimulate and appear to speed up thinking. Often abused by people wishing to stay awake.
Anal intercourse/ sex:	Insertion of a man's penis into the anus of a man, woman, or child. Even in adults can cause slight bleeding.
Antibodies:	Substance produced by white cells to destroy germs.
Asymptomatic:	Person feels well.
Autologous blood transfusion:	Giving and storing your own blood, which is given back to you after an operation.
Azidothymidine:	Anti-viral drug being evaluated (see also AZT).
Bestiality:	Intercourse between an animal and a man or woman. More common these days than many realise.
Biopsy:	Taking a tiny piece of tissue for examination under the microscope.
Bi-sexual:	Someone attracted sexually to both men and women.
Body-positive:	Someone who has sero-converted HIV (see also HIV).
Bone marrow:	Hollow red spongy core of human bones. It makes blood cells. Can be affected by many anti-AIDS or anti-cancer drugs and by radiotherapy.
Bronchoalveolar lavage:	Collecting fiuids from inside the lung. Used to try and identify cause of pneumonias in people with AIDS.
Bronchoscopy:	Insertion of a tube, with a special tiny camera on the end, down the windpipe into the lungs to look and take samples. Patient sedated first.
Buddies:	System of friendships and caregivers for those with AIDS who may be feeling extremely vulnerable, lonely, isolated, rejected, and depressed. It has been very successful in providing support and care.
Buggery:	Placing of a man's penis in a boy or man's rectum.
Cannabis:	Leaves of plant smoked like tobacco for mood-altering and relaxing effects.
CAT scan:	Special computerised X-ray machine that can produce excellent pictures of brain, lung, or abdomen for particular purposes. Huge and expensive. Not available everywhere.
Cerebrospinal fluid:	Fluid removed during lumbar puncture. Normally bathes brain and spinal cord. Can be infected in meningitis. See also Lumbar puncture.
Co-factor:	An additional feature that may influence infection—usually making it more likely.
Cold turkey:	Addict may experience severe symptoms with shaking and aches all over as he withdraws suddenly from the drug.
Coming out:	For a homosexual this means being open and honest about

	his or her sexual preferences and lifestyle. Being unashamed.
Condom:	Sheath made of latex rubber or animal membrane designed to fit over the erect penis during intercourse to collect seminal fluid and reduce the risk of pregnancy. Also reduces risk of HIV infection greatly (by 85 per cent) but not completely.
Co-trimoxazole (Septrin):	Antibiotic used to treat *pneumocystis carinii* chest infections.
Crack:	Cocaine. May depress immunity still further.
Cryptosporidium:	Common infection in AIDS.
Cum:	Slang for seminal fluid.
Cytomegalovirus:	(CMV) Common infection in AIDS.
Dimethylfluorornithine:	Antibiotic used to treat pneumocystis chest infections.
Dope:	Loose term used to cover a wide variety of drugs taken for mood-altering properties as part of addiction or abuse.
Doubling time:	Length of time for the number of cases of AIDS to double.
Downers:	Barbiturates and other sedatives taken to slow someone down after taking amphetamines. See also Amphetamines.
Encephalitis:	Inflammation of the brain due to infection.
Factor VIII:	Substance required by haemophiliacs (blood extract).
Fibre optic:	Name given to cameras used in endoscopy and bronchoscopy which are in fact made of thousands of tiny glass fibres. See also Bronchoscopy.
Fix:	Dose of drug given into vein.
Flashback:	Reliving of a previous LSD trip. See also LSD.
Foscarnet:	Anti-viral drug being evaluated.
Gallium lung scans:	Test used to confirm pneumocystis chest infection.
Gay:	Alternative name for homosexual (recent use), usually of someone has 'come out'. See also Come out.
Hashish:	Cannabis. See also Cannabis.
Hepatitis B:	Blood-borne disease caused by virus. Can be caught in similar ways to HIV, but much more infectious. Causes liver damage which can be fatal. Two thousand cases in UK in 1987 (increasing).
Herpes Simplex type 1:	Causes sores around mouth: 'cold sores'.
Herpes Simplex type 2:	Causes painful sores in the genital/anal areas. May increase risk of cervical cancer. Highly infectious when activated.
Heterosexual:	Someone whose sexual preference is for someone of the opposite sex.
High:	Mental state of an addict after taking drugs.

Homosexual: Someone whose sexual preference is for someone of the same sex.

Immunoglobulin: Antibody. See also Antibody.

Immuno-suppression: Body's natural defences against disease reduced: white cells and antibodies are less effective or less in quantity.

Inosine pranobex: See Isoprinosine.

Interferon: Substance made by infected cells. Protects against further viruses entering cell. Can be manufactured. Has been used in chemotherapy.

Interleukin 2: Substance usually produced by T4 white cells. Being evaluated as an anti-AIDS drug.

Isoprinosine: Drug tried with little success.

Johnny: See Condom.

Joint: Marijuana cigarette containing cannabis. See also Cannabis.

Lesser AIDS: See ARC.

Lumbar puncture: Insertion of a needle in the lower back under local anaesthetic to remove a sample of fluid from the fluid covering the brain and spinal cord. Usually to try and find cause of a new infection.

Lymph node: Small gland usually too small to feel. Swollen in infections. Filters out germs preventing them from reaching the blood. Full of white cells.

Lymphocyte: White cell—part of body's defence against infection. Two types: B cells produce antibodies. T cells sometimes kill germs directly, others help B cells prepare the right antibody. The T4 lymphocytes are the ones infected by HIV.

Lymphoma: Unusual kind of cancer involving white cells of the body.

Mainlining: Injection of drugs directly into a vein by an addict. This is carried in one big amount through the lungs and into the brain via arteries. The travel time from arm to brain is about one minute. After ten minutes the drug is then diluted throughout the entire body, but the addict has experienced a huge 'kick' or 'buzz' from only a relatively small dose.

The body has virtually no defences against germs entering the blood directly so dirty needles make addicts very ill. If shared, the needles transfer blood and HIV from one addict to another.

Many addicts die from an overdose. They buy heroin 'cut' with anything ranging from salt and sugar to chalk. They measure out the mixture which may have very little heroin in it. One day they meet a dealer who sells them the pure drug. They measure out the same volume and it kills them. The drug overdose stops their breathing for about one to three minutes after the injection. Brain damage may start three minutes after that.

Meningitis: Inflammation of the surface of the brain due to infection.

Methisoprinol: See Isoprinosine.

Neonatal: Pertaining to a newborn baby.

Nitrites: Drugs taken to increase sexual arousal. There is a worrying association between use of nitrites and developing Kaposi's sarcoma. Nitrites certainly damage immunity which can be lethal in someone infected with HIV.

Oesophagus: Tube connecting mouth to stomach.

Oral sex: Genital contact with the mouth of a sexual partner. Dangerous if one partner infected.

Pentamidine: Antibiotic used to treat pneumocystis pneumonia.

Pleural effusion: Water between the lung and the chest wall, caused by infection or cancer. Can reduce the amount of air in the lung and cause shortness of breath.

Pneumocystis carinii: Unusual fungus, causing chronic severe lung infections in people with AIDS. Usually treated with septrin/co-trimoxazole, or pentamidine.

Pneumothorax: Collapse of a lung. Can cause chest pain and sudden shortness of breath. Usually gets better quickly by itself, but may require treatment. Sometimes follows pneumocystis infection or a bronchoscopy.

Poppers: Slang for nitrites (see also).

Pre-AIDS: See ARC.

Prodromal AIDS: See ARC.

Q Substance: Trichosanthrin—drug under trial.

Retrovirus: A virus which makes new DNA code from its own RNA using the enzyme reverse transcriptase. HIV is an example.

Reverse transcriptase: Enzyme used to make DNA in a cell nucleus as a carbon copy of RNA from virus. Many AIDS drugs try to prevent this enzyme from working.

Ribavirin: Anti-viral drug being evaluated.

Seminal fluid: Fluid produced by a man when sexually aroused. Contains sperm.

Septicaemia: Situation where a (bacterial) infection has spread from a localised part of the body into the bloodstream. The result is someone who feels very unwell, may have a high temperature, and may be shaking uncontrollably.

Septrin: See Co-trimoxazole.

Sero-conversion: Time when person begins to carry antibodies in his or her blood indicating HIV infection.

Sero-positive: Antibodies to HIV present in the blood.

Sex-change operation: Mutilating operation to cut off a man's penis and testicles. A section of bowel is cut out and turned into a blind pouch.

This is sewn into the skin at a point roughly where a woman's vagina would be expected to be. The result is an opening which can function as a crude vagina. Several such operations are carried out in London each week. It is a major procedure because it involves cutting intestines with risks of infection. It also requires a long anaesthetic. By psychiatrists people are referred to surgeons. Medically the person is regarded as mentally ill, he has a delusion that he is a woman born by accident into a male body. Because psychiatrists sometimes cannot alter this belief, one or two suggest altering appearance. Stage one is giving female hormones to a man so his breasts grow to a woman's size. Stage two is amputation of his penis and the rest. Sex is determined by genetic code as a 'fact of life'. The sex change is a crude cosmetic attempt to enable a man to pass himself off as a woman—especially in bed.

The results can be grotesque: a fifty-five-year old huge rugby player with coarse features and beard with large breasts and a missing penis. The beard needs shaving every day. Removal of male hormones does not change your build or facial hair. In people from the East who often have small build and minimal facial hair, the operation can have staggering results. I remember a man who had succeeded in being married to another unsuspecting man for several years. He came over to the United Kingdom again because the gut pouch was narrowing so sex was becoming impossible. A further operation was carried out.

Many doctors, of whatever faith or no faith, consider the procedure to be unethical and wrong. Since when has it been right to reinforce someone's lost grip on reality by agreeing to mutilate the person especially when the procedure could kill? This is not a minor procedure. If someone went to a psychiatrist convinced that cockroaches were living in his left leg, causing him terrible pains as they ate up his body, do you think it would be good medical care to cut his leg off on the basis that it would probably make him more content?

A friend of mine was worried recently because as a junior doctor one of his patients told him he had changed his mind yet again about 'having it done'. The man already had breasts, had posed successfully as a woman for some months (a condition of the operation), but said he now had had second thoughts. My friend decided not to sign him up for the operation and got into trouble with a senior colleague. The operation was done and the man had a big reaction afterward. He could not remember if he had agreed to it or not. As many as thirty out of one hundred people are dissatisfied, asking for reversal (impossible) or committing suicide.

A family doctor I know broke partnership with a colleague in her practice after an attractive eighteen-year-old girl had walked into her surgery: 'Don't you remember me?' she exclaimed. 'I'm Roger, you remember?' This had been the adolescent sixteen-year-old boy who was confused about his sexuality. The doctor violently objected to her colleague. Surely to send a teenager for an opinion about a sex change operation was a terrible thing. It cannot be reversed. You cannot replace a man's genitalia any more than a woman's womb.

Medicine cannot alter the code of all your cells, only mutilate your appearance in order to allow deception. A friend of mine (male) was shocked one day to discover that he had been dating another man who was taking female hormones. He felt deceived, cheated, and angry with the person and his doctor. He had been thinking of marriage. He was a devout Christian.

Shingles: Painful skin condition caused by chicken-pox virus.

Shooting gallery: Place where addicts meet together to inject drugs. Part of the culture which makes the habit even harder to break is the whole ritual of drug abuse: meeting together, mixing the drug, drawing up the syringe, and injecting, often everyone using the same needle. People often feel safer with others—in case someone overdoses or has a bad trip (on LSD).

Snorting: Sniffing cocaine or heroin up the nose.

Speed: See Amphetamines.

Sperm: Tadpole-shaped organisms consisting of a single human cell containing half of a complete genetic code. The other half is contained in a human egg.

Spermicide: Chemicals which prevent tails of sperm moving, and therefore prevent fertilisation of an egg. Spermicides containing non-oxynol may give added protection against AIDS when used with a condom.

Spunk: Slang for seminal fluid.

Suramin: Anti-viral drug with slight effect on HIV but having serious side-effects.

Surrogate mother: A woman bearing another woman's child. Usually result of a test-tube baby conceived using someone else's egg and donated sperm, implanted in her womb. The developing baby uses her body as a 'hotel' during development. Hiring a womb like this raises enormous emotional and ethical issues.

Systemic infection: Affecting the whole body.

Test-tube baby: Baby conceived by placing a drop of a man's seminal fluids onto a glass slide containing a human egg. When fertilisation occurs, the egg starts to divide, and this is checked under the microscope. At a certain critical stage the rapidly developing embryo is placed in the womb of the woman.

Obtaining eggs is far more difficult than obtaining semen. Because success rates are low, women are given drugs to make the ovary produce several eggs at once—normally it produces one a month. The woman then has an operation to collect the eggs. As many as twelve eggs are exposed to sperm and usually three or four are put in the womb. Because embryos often die without settling in the womb the result can be no baby, one baby, or twins. Occasionally triplets or quadruplets are born.

What do we do with the other developing babies? At the moment they are used for experiments. The first experiment tries to see if they can be kept alive for longer in the laboratory. The second kind of experiment exposes them to all sorts of chemicals to see what happens. These experiments happen every day in the United Kingdom despite several attempts by medical personnel to stop them.

The way to stop it is to fertilise only the number of eggs that could safely be placed inside a woman. Abortion has so cheapened the life of a baby in the womb that many cannot see the issue of experimenting on these 'things' at all. We distance ourselves by using scientific terms like morula, foetus, or embryo when medically there is no distinction between them. What is the difference between life after an hour, a week, a month, or ten years? Logically, there is none.

Thrush: Fungal infection of mouth, throat, gut, or skin caused by *candida albicans*.

Toxoplasmosis: Common infection in AIDS.

Transmission: Passing of infection from one person to another.

Trip: Experience of an addict after drug taking.

Venereal disease: Sexually transmitted disease.

Virus: Bag of protein containing genetic code, capable of infecting a cell and instructing it to make new viruses.

Withdrawal (of drug addict): Stopping drug supply to someone who is dependent. Can produce symptoms such as severe shakes and cramps (see also Cold turkey).

Works: Needle and syringe used by an addict. The habit of flushing remaining drug out of the syringe by drawing back your own blood leaves gross contamination of the syringe as well as the needle, and increases the risk of getting HIV infection enormously as the works are passed around.

Notes

Chapter 1 The Extent of the Nightmare

1. *Morbidity and Mortality Weekly Report* (United States), 30 (1981): 305–308.
2. Ten people are ill with pre-AIDS/AIDS-related complex (ARC) for each person with full-blown AIDS. However, figures quoted are always for AIDS. *Medical Clinics of North America*, 70 (1986): 693–705.
3. Rees estimated 2.5 million infected in the United States by as early as 1984. *Nature* (United Kingdom), 326 (16 April 1987): 636.
4. Dr Robert Gallo co-discoverer of HIV. *Scientific American*, 265 (1987): 39–48. His discovery disputed though—see p. 60.
5. Major damage to the immune system can be detected in two out of ten peole infected after only two years. After only five years, half those infected have abnormal immune systems. After seven years two-thirds of those infected have developed AIDS or are unwell with early AIDS (*AIDSFILE* [June 1987]). But this is a slow virus. Other slow viruses do not cause disease until ten, twenty, or even forty years after infection. *Nature*, 326 (1987): 636. In Germany, only thirty out of 377 infected people were still well after three years of infection. Half of those infected had developed early signs (swollen glands) after only a year. Of those with any damage to their immune systems, half had already gone on to develop full-blown AIDS in two years. There may be a reason why this particular group is deteriorating so fast (*Nature*, 324 [1986]: 1999). German authorities have predicted seventy-five out of one hundred infected people developing full blown AIDS in seven years (*Deutsche Medizinische Wochenschrift*, 3:40 [1986]: 1540). San Francisco studies predict 75 per cent developing AIDS in ten years. Press reports March 1990.
6. *AIDS Weekly Surveillance Report* (United States: 1987).
7. *USA Public Health Reports,* 102 (1986): 341.
8. 'Epidemiolgoy of AIDS in the United States' (excellent review), *Scientific American*, (October 1988): 52–59.
9. Isolated case reports from 1962 to date; but only recognised as such in 1980s *Scandinavian Journal of Infectious Diseases,* 5 (1987): 511–517; also *Canadian Medical Association Journal*, 137:7 (1987): 637.
10. Personal communications. Information from Africa is politically sensitive.

Workers have to keep their mouths shut or face imprisonment or deportation. Often the source or even the country cannot be identified, to protect doctors and scientists. Uganda has led the way with openness, admitting to one in eight of all adults infected (1 million)—1990 figures.

11. Up to 68 per cent of barmaids were infected in Southwest Uganda. *AIDS*, 1;4 (1987): 223–227.
12. Personal communications. (See endnote no. 10.)
13. Four out of ten men (twenty to thirty years old) in Lusaka hospital (Zambia) were infected. *International Herald Tribune* (4 July 1987; also 5 July 1987). Unofficial reports of 60 per cent of Zimbabwe troops infected.
14. Predictions of which agricultural systems will be worst affected by AIDS labour loss. *New Scientist*, 117 (14 January 1988): 34–35.
15. Personal communications. (See endnote no.10.)
16. *Annales de la Société Belge de Médicine Tropicale,* 66: 3 (1986): 345–350. See Chapter 4, p. 75.
17. Worst prediction is that seven out of ten of all men and women will be infected in Central Africa in ten years' time (*AIDS-Forschung*, 2, 1 [1987]: 5–25). Population of the whole continent was 555 million in 1985 (Commonwealth Institute, United Kingdom).
18. It is hard to understand how low development agencies place AIDS.
19. *World Health Forum 4:3 (1988): 384. Uganda Report, 3:2 (1989): 79–85.*
20. World Health Organisation figures July 1990, *New England Journal of Medicine*, 319: 5 (1988): 302–303, BMA/RGN conference, March 1990.
21. *Lancet*, 2 (1981): 1339.
22. *Lancet*, 1 (1985): 1261–1262. (Clinic for sexually-transmitted diseases.)
23. Proportions of homosexual men attending clinics for sexually-transmitted diseases who are infected with HIV have been recorded as high as thirty-five out of one hundred (*British Medical Journal*, 290 [1985]: 1176). However, this may be artificially high because less promiscuous groups may not be attending the clinics, and people developing symptoms related to AIDS are included.
24. Men with more than forty-nine male partners a year. *New Scientist*, (26 March 1987): 55.
25. See chapter 4, page 78.
26. *American Journal of Public Health*, 77 (1987): 578–581.
27. Each prostitute may have sex with several thousand people a year. (see Chapter 7, page 132; Chapter 4, pages 75–78.) 1% heterosexuals reported. *British Medical Journal* 298 (February 18, 1989): 419–422.
28. 60,000 quoted in *Independent* (9 January 1987). Rees estimated possibly 110,000 in the United Kingdom were infected as early as 1985. *Nature* , 326 (1987): 343–345. Most people think these were too high.
29. Government's Chief Nursing Officer speaking at the Royal College of Nursing conference on AIDS in the community, January 1987. Voluntary testing is actually identifying around two hundred new infections out

of the estimated total new infections of up to fifteen hundred each month.

30. *AIDS Bulletin*, 3 (1988): 62.
31. Personal communication. Many of these people are married.
32. *Observer* (London: 10 May 1987).
33. *Lancet*, 2 (1986): 814 (nurse). *Lancet*, 1 (1983): 925 (surgeon). *New York Times* (6 June 1987), (dentist). Total of thirty-four health care workers reported infected (worldwide totals) through their work. *British Medical Journal*, 297 (1988): 244. Risk from needlestick injury less than 1:200.
34. See Chapter 5, page 87 for discussions of risks.
35. *Annals of Internal Medicine*, 106: 2 (1987):, 244–245 (kidney transplant). *Lancet*, 1 (1987): 983 (skin donor).
36. House of Commons debate March 6 1990.
37. *Today* (29 April 1987).
38. *Atlantic Monthly* (February 1987): 48.
39. *The Times* (6 January 1987).
40. *The Times* (13 July 1987). Clifford Longley: 'Since 1981 the church has continued to recruit to the ministry men who are homosexual and they have continued to engage, if discreetly, in homosexual activities.'
41. Front page of *Sun* newspaper (London: 9 July 1987). Source: the Rev. Tony Higton, Rector of Hawkwell, Essex.
42. Andrew Walker *Restoring the Kingdom* (Hodder and Stoughton, 1986). Contains extensive review of these new churches. See also *Going by the Book*, BBC2 (27 August 1987).
43. 'ABC of Sexually Transmitted Diseases,' *British Medical Journal*, special edition (book of reprints, 1984): 1.
44. A famous United States Army war poster was of a prostitute walking with Hitler on one arm and the Japanese Emperor on the other. The caption read: 'VD (venereal disease) worst of the three.'
45. 'ABC of Sexually Transmitted Diseases,' 1.
46. See Chapter 6, pages 107–117.
47. *Reviews of Infectious Diseases*, 9:6 (1987): 1102–1108.
48. Clumeck's famous letter to *Lancet* in 1983. Many still dispute that HIV first infected people in Africa. What is the evidence? Old blood samples dated from the 1960s from people in Central Africa have been found positive when tested for HIV infection (*New Scientist* [22 January 1987]). One sample, dated 1959, was also positive. However, an early AIDS case was recently confirmed in a sailor from Manchester dated 1959. It seems his wife also died of AIDS. *The Independent* 6 July 1990. Some of the African results have been questioned: traces of malaria infection, and other things, can sometimes confuse the testing. The local monkey population is well-known for being infected with viruses which are very similar to those producing AIDS. Nearly one-third of some species are infected in some areas. 'Field study among African Primates' (*Microbiology and*

Immunology, 30: 4 [1986]: 315–321; also 'AIDS in an African Context,' *Nature* [1986]: 324. Spread from monkeys to man could have been from bites, bestiality (common in all countries of the world including the United Kingdom), or the practice of certain African tribes inoculating people with monkey blood as part of a fertility rite (*Lancet*, 1 [1987]: 1498–1499; also *New Scientist* [16 July 1987]). One report has suggested monkey-human spread was the result of eating green monkeys! AIDS seems common in areas where consumption is high (*Guardian* [19 February 1987]). There is also evidence of AIDS in the United States as early as 1968 and possibly as early as 1958 (1988 reports from Washington University and the Medical University of South Carolina). Wherever it first came from, there is little idea as to why it has apparently spread so much faster in Africa than elsewhere. There is no genetic susceptibility (*AIDS*, 1: 4 [1987]: 258–259; also *Lancet*, 1 [23 April 1988]: 936)—a previous paper's figures were wrongly added. Spread is more likely where other sex diseases result in untreated genital ulcerations. This is common in Africa due to inadequate facilities. Excellent summary of origins discussion: *Scientific American*, October 1988, 44–51.

49. This sounds terrible, but New York City now has over twenty thousand cases of AIDS and five hundred thousand infected (estimate), according to the *AIDS Weekly Surveillance Report* (United States: 1987). Gay behaviour changed dramatically in San Francisco between 1983 and 1986, although heterosexual teenagers continue to take big risks (*New Scientist* [7 January 1988]: 36–37; also *American Journal of Public Health*, 78: 4 [1988]: 460–461). Elsewhere in the United States gay behaviour changes are variable or nonexistent.
50. Personal communication.
51. 'AIDS Has Created a New Form of Bereavement,' *Canadian Medical Association Journal*, 136: 2 (1987): 194.
52. Five cases of mental illness resulting from fears of catching AIDS have been reported ('AIDS-Phobia,' *British Journal of Psychology*, 150 [1987]: 412–413; Also *British Journal of Psychology*, 152 [March 1988]: 424–475). However doctors must take care not to miss true disease: a Boston doctor has been sued for $750,000 damages by a woman whom he misdiagnosed as an asthmatic with imaginary symptoms when she had an AIDS-related pneumonia. *The Times* (21 February 1988).
53. *AIDSFILE*, 1: 3 (1968): 1.
54. United Kingdom. Financial consequences are far more catastrophic if you are ill in the United States.
55. *Daily Telegraph* (London: 11 February 1987; also 2 February 1987); also *Sunday Telegraph* (London: 15 February 1987).
56. AIDS Newsletter 5. Bureau of Hygiene and Tropical Diseases (February 1987).
57. *Star* newspaper (London). Complaint to Press Council dismissed as 'in

public interest' (*The Times* [20 July 1987]). From 1985 *Dan-Air* only took female cabin staff for this reason. This was outlawed by the Equal Opportunities Commission in 1987. *The Times* (3 February 1987).

58. *Daily Telegraph* (London: 11 February 1987; also 14 February 1987); also *Sunday Telegraph* (London: 15 February 1987).
59. Personal communication from the person who was thinking of introducing it to prevent collapse of the service.
60. *American Journal of Public Health*, 76 (1968): 1325–30; also 'AIDS Stress Health Care in San Francisco,' *Science* (USA), 235)1987): 964.
61. Middlesex, St Stephens, and St Mary's Hospitals report to the Social Services Committee, *Independent* (5 March 1987).
62. *Bulletin of the New York Academy of Medicine* 64: 2)1988): 175–183.
63. *International Herald Tribune* (23 August 1988): 3.
64. *The Times* (14 July 1988).
65. Personal communication.
66. Editorial, *Nature*, 334 (11 August 198): 457.
67. 'Understanding AIDS' leaflet mailed May-June, 1988. *American Journal of Preventative Medicine*, 4:4 (1988): 239–240 gives useful background.
68. Several have died without ever developing so-called AIDS in San Francisco (personal communication).
69. *International Herald Tribune* (2 September 1988): 4.
70. The new AIDS definitions are broader now and have resulted in an increase of 19 per cent in total numbers meeting the grade (*Journal of the American Medical Association*, 259: 15 [1988]; 2235; also *Lancet*, 1 [5 March 1988]: 520–521). Details of new definitions in *Morbidity and Mortality Weekly Report*, 36 (14 August 1987). See Table on page 71.
71. See Chapter 3, page 68. 11% of AIDS patients survive more than three years.
72. Personal communication.
73. Example: 'The virus ... is extremely fragile and can only live momentarily outside body fluids.' *London Lighthouse* (AIDS hospice) *Newletter*, 2 (April 1987).
74. *Journal of the American Medical Association*, *(JAMA)*, 255: 14 (1986): 1887–1891.
75. LAV/HTVL-III. Causative agent of AIDS and related conditions. Revised guidelines (June 1986). The DHSS is now two departments.
76. Personal communication.
77. *Lancet*, 2 (1987): 166. See page 93.
78. It has also been pointed out recently that figures for known HIV positive people may be gross underestimates because so many are being tested at private clinics which do not send out statistics. Also the HIV over-the-counter home-testing kits—not illegal in the United Kingdom—will make matters worse. *Doctor* (18 August 1988).

79. Several cases in older people missed recently in the United Kingdom. *Independent* (16 September 1988); also *British Medical Journal.*
80. Dr Anna McCormick of United Kingdom Office of Population Censuses and Surveys detected 887 more deaths than expected in single men fifteen to fifty-four years old from 1984–1987. On inspection of records only half were diagnosed as AIDS cases although most of the rest died of conditions often causing AIDS deaths. She concluded that recorded United Kingdom AIDS deaths may be only half the story. *British Medical Journal*, 296 (1988): 1289–1292.
81. *Journal of the American Medical Association*, 257 (1987): 1727.
82. This is a cheap, reliable way to confirm AIDS diagnosis in someone who has all the appearances of it. Because almost everyone in Africa has had some slight exposure to TB, nearly everyone reacts positively to the special skin test. A sign of AIDS is that the person's body fails to produce the skin bump usually seen. The test is cheap and widely available in Africa, unlike AIDS testing kits. Personal communication.
83. President Kaunda's son (Zambia)—*The Times* (London) (5 October 1987).
84. Dissenting voice: 'Point of view,' *Lancet*, (1987): 2906–207. Article questions if situation is as bad as feared—based on a personal tour.
85. Unofficial reports of 6 in 100 newborn babies in Soweto testing positive. Personal communication.
86. *AIDS Newsletter*, 2: 11 (1987). Bureau of Hygiene and Tropical Diseases.
87. *Sunday Express*, (London: 12 July 1987).
88. *Independent* (16 February, 1987).

Chapter 2 What's So Special about a Virus?

1. A scientist called Duesberg has suggested that AIDS is not caused by HIV but by some other agent. He is regarded as an eccentric and his original paper has been heavily criticised as being full of inaccuracies (*Cancer Research*, 47 [1987]: 1199–1220). To read both sides of a confusing debate see *New Scientist*, 118 (28 April 1988): 34–35; also (5 May 1988): 32–33. Also *Science* 243 (1989): 733.
2. Excellent review articles: *Scientific American*, 255 (1966): 78–88; also 256 (1987): 38–48.
3. A number of bills have been presented by members of Parliament to limit experimentation on human embryos. None has succeeded in becoming law so far, due to lack of government support. See 'test-tube babies' in the glossary of terms.
4. A number of experiments are described in *Nature* (6 August 1987): 12.
5. Examples simplified enormously.

6. *Journal of the American Medical Association*, 259: 20 (1988): 3037–3038.
7. *New Scientist*, 113 (26 March 1987): 36–37.
8. Excellent article: 'AIDS in 1988,' *Scientific American*, 259 (4 October 1988): 25–32.
9. *Scientific American*, 259 (October 1988): 34–42.
10. *New Scientist*, 113 (26 March 1987): 46–51.
11. Ibid.
12. Thirty-nine minor variations of HIV found in two patients. *Nature*, 334 (4 August 1988): 440–444.
13. 'HIV-2 infection,' *Lancet*, 1 (1987): 223; also 'An Unexpected New Virus' (HBLV), *Lancet*, 2 (1986): 1430–1431.
14. These are viruses with differences in shape and character.
15. *Nature*, 325 (1987): 765.
16. Ibid.
17. This has recently been done. *Nature*, 331 (1988): 76–78, 15, 79.
18. Further reading: 'Is a Vaccine Against AIDS Possible?', *Vaccine*, 6: 1 (1988): 3–5; 'Strategies for an AIDS Vaccine,' 233 (United States: 1986): 1149–1153; 'Problems with AIDS Vaccines,' *Nature*, 324 (1986): 304; 'Prospects for an AIDS Vaccine,' PHLS *Microbiology Digest*, vol. 4, no. 2 (1987): 26–30.
19. *Nature*, 330 (24/31 December 1987): 702–703.
20. Proceedings of National Academy of Sciences of U.S.A., 85:23 (1988): 9234–9257.
21. *Federal Register* (19 March 1987). New legislation relaxing the rules. Despite this chimpanzees, which are commonly used in AIDS research, could easily become extinct because of over-use in laboratories testing AIDS drugs and vaccines. ATLA *(Alternatives to Laboratory Animals)*, 15: 3 (1988): 176–179. Zidovudine (AZT) resistance described in Wellcome press release, March 1989. Also *New England Journal of Medicine* 320:9 (1989): 594–595.
22. Ibid.
23. House of Lords question by Baroness Seear to government spokesman (*Hansard*, 29 June 1987).
24. Testing can often be difficult due to issues surrounding certain ethical objections and problems related to finding willing volunteers. See *New Scientist* (12 November 1988): 26–27.
25. 'Imminent Marketing of AZT Raises Problems,' *Science*, 235 (United States: 1987): 1462–1463.
26. 'Will an AIDS Vaccine Bankrupt the Company That Makes It?', *Science*, 233 (1986): 1035.
27. Settlement on AIDS Finally Reached Between USA and Pasteur,' *Nature*, 326 (1987): 533, row continues however, *Nature*, 345 (1990): 104.
28. Sales were worth $65 million up to 27 February 1988 with profits of $6 million after development costs. Political and social pressures—'AZT

should be free'—in the United States led to a 20 per cent drop. Wellcome's total profits were up by 35 per cent in 1988 because of AZT and another drug used in AIDS teatment (Zovirax), *The Times* (11 November 1988). The Queen's Award for technological achievement was granted to Wellcome for AZT, *The Times* (21 April 1990).

29. 'Testing an AIDS vaccine may be harder than inventing one,' *Scientific American*, 258: 2 (1988): 18–19. Some think it likely that vaccines will be tried out in Africa without permission from governments or individuals. *International Herald Tribune*, (22 September 1988): 7.
30. Personal communication (May 1990).
31. *Canadian Medical Association Journal*, 137: 10 (1987): 932–933.
32. 'AIDS Prevention Trade Booming,' *Journal of Commerce* (international edition) (9 May 1988): 1.
33. See page 30.
34. Ibid.
35. See Chapter 6.

Chapter 3 When the Cells Start to Die

1. *Journal of the American Medical Association*, 257: 10 (1987): 1327. It seems people are much less infectious when they are well.
2. See endnotes for Chapter 1, page 245.
3. One study showed thirteen out of one hundred had gone on to develop full-blown AIDS in two years (*British Medical Journal*,) 294 [1987]: 868–869). But other studies are not so optimistic – see page 38.
4. 'AIDS and the Dentist,' *British Dental Journal*, 162: 10 (1987): 375; also *New Scientist* (19 February 1987): 19.
5. In people without AIDS, antibiotics start the job and the body does the rest. If the immune system is damaged, it is sometimes extremely difficult to get rid of the germ completely. An example is syphilis where it seems that prolonged high dose antibiotics are required to prevent relapse. *New England Journal of Medicine*, vol. 316 (1987): 1569–1572; 1587–1589; 1600–1601.
6. *Respiratory Disease in Practice* (October/November 1988).
7. 'AIDS Not Gentle on the Mind'—excellent review article, *New Scientist*, 113 (26 March 1987): 38–39.
8. *AIDSFILE*, 1: 3 (1986): 1.
9. Chief Neurosurgeon in San Francisco gave a verbal report on a series of post-mortems of people who died of AIDS. Each showed damage to the brain.
10. *Science*, 233 (United States: 1986): 1089–1093.
11. *Cell*, 47:3 (1986): 1.

13. *Pediatrics*, 78:4 (1986): 678–687. The mean lifetime cost (in patient) per child with AIDS in New York is $90,347. *Journal of the American Medical Association*, 260: 13 (1988, 260): 1901–1905.
14. The spinal cord, for example (*British Medical Journal*, 294 [1987]: 143–144). Brain damage may overtake pneumonia and cancers as the main cause of death, according to Dr Richard Johnson, Chairman of the Department of Neurology at Johns Hopkins Medical School, Baltimore, Maryland (November 1988).
15. *Pediatric Infectious Disease Journal*, 7: 5 (1988): 561–571.
16. ARC stands for: AIDS-related complex.
17. Further reading and colour illustrations: *British Medical Journal*, 294 (1987): 29–32.
18. *Lancet*, 1 (1987): 280–281.
19. *Journal of Infectious Diseases*, 157: 5 (1988): 1044–1047. Other data on survival times: *Lancet*, (6 April 1988): 880.
20. *Quarterly Journal of Medicine*, 67: 254 (1988): 473–486.
21. Ibid.
22. *Journal of the American Medical Association*, 257 (1987): 3066.
23. *American Journal of Diseases of Children*, 140: 12 (1986): 1241–1244.

Chapter 4 How People Become Infected

1. Federal official Dr Antonia Novella speaking (18 December 1988). AIDS is now number nine in the list of causes of death in United States for children from one to four years of age. (Report of United States Health and Human Services, December 1988).
2. See Chapter 6.
3. Dr Jacquie Mok, consultant pediatrician at Edinburgh City Hospital is now facing a huge problem with already seventy 'positive' babies to follow up. The mothers are usually drug addicts. *Independent* (6 July 1987).
4. 'AIDS and Human Milk Bank Closures,' *Lancet*, 1 (1987): 1092–1093.
5. *Microtransfusions—one in five of some children infected (1990).*
6. *Daily Telegraph*, (London: 19 March 1987).
7. *Journal of the American Medical Association*, 256: 22 (1986), 3094.
8. *The Times* (30 April 1987); possibly two more *The Times* (1 August 1987).
9. *Journal of Pediatrics*, 112: 6 (1988): 1005–1007.
10. *Pediatrics*, 1987, 80: 4 (1987): 561–564.
11. *British Medical Journal*, 294 (1987): 389–390.
12. AIDS, 1: 1 (1987): 39–44.
13. *Journal of Infectious Diseases*, 155:4 (1987): 828.
14. Five million iv drug users in the world (UN estimate, 31 March 1990).

15. *Guardian*, (6 July 1987).
16. *British Medical Journal*, 294 (1987): 389–390.
17. One in every two hundred fifty people in Merseyside uses heroin or similar drugs. This explosion of drug abuse began only five years ago. However, most of the addicts in Merseyside sniff herion and do not inject. *British Journal of Addiction*, vol. 82 (1987): 147–57.
18. *Journal of the American Medical Association*, 259:15 (1988): 859.
19. *Guardian* (6 July 1987).
20. *British Medical Journal*, 294 (1987): 571–572; also 297 (1988): 859.
21. Scottish police inspector at conference in Peebles (April 1987).
22. Chalk, being white, is often mixed with heroin by dealers to cheat drug users.
23. *Lancet* 1 (1982): 1983–1087.
24. *International Herald Tribune*. High priced prostitues—only one in seventy-eight infected compared to 9–21 per cent of those on the street. In Glasgow, Scotland, 768 of prostitutes are injecting or have injected drugs. *Communicable Diseases Unit* (Scotland: 14 November 1988).
25. *Journal of the American Medical Association*, 257: 3 (1987): 321–325.
26. *Journal of the American Medical Association*, 258: 4 (1987): 474.
27. *New Scientist*, (26 March 1987): 55. However, rectal trauma (pushing a fist and possibly a forearm into the anus, pre-sex enemas, scarring, fistulas, or fissures) and receptive anal intercourse are high risk factors also. *American Journal of Epidemiology*, 138:4 (1987): 508–577.
28. Ibid.
29. See endnotes, Chapter 1, page 245.
30. *American Journal of Public Health*, 177 (1987): 578–581.
31. *Science* (United States: 1987): 382.
32. Personal communication in San Francisco.
33. The other prison risk is widespread drug abuse. *The Times* headlines (27 July 1987); *British Medical Journal*, 297 (8 October 1988): 873–874.
34. 'Could a Prisoner Sue the Authorities for Inadequate Protection?', *AIDS-Forschung*, 2: 2 (1987): 52, 55.
35. All infected prisoners are being isolated in Brixton prison in a new unit for protection of and from other prisoners. *The Times* (22 April 1987).
36. Charing Cross Hospital lecture on sexually-transmitted diseases.
37. *New Scientist* (26 March 1987): 56.
38. 'Male Rape: Breaking the Silence on a Taboo Subject,' 278 rapes of men by men in Southeast England in 1986. *The Listener* (23 July 1987).
39. *New Scientist* (26 March 1987): 56–57.
40. Personal communication.
41. *New Scientist* (26 March 1987): 56–57.
42. *Shanti* is a sanskrit word meaning peace.
43. Christopher Spence, director of London Lighthouse (AIDS hospice),

'AIDS and the Wind of Change,' *Leading Lights* newsletter (April 1987): 3–4.

44. Dr Mann (World Health Organisation) at conference in Washington, D.C., (June 1987).
45. *Independent* (4 Februray 1987).
46. *Financial Times* (11 April 1987).
47. *Guardian* (16 February 1988): 2.
48. Chief Executive magazine survey reported in *Daily Telegraph* (9 March 1987).
49. For example, Jeffrey Archer, member of Parliament, and the prostitute libel case. He won but they won: a destroyed political career. All because they suggested he had spent a night with a prostitute.
50. Three risk factors for transmission from an infected man to a woman: STD in last 5 years, partner with AIDS, and anal intercourse. Transmission occured in 27% of 155 heterosexual couples overall and 67% in those with more than two risk factors. *British Medical Journal*, 298 (1989): 411–415.
51. The diocesan AIDS office in San Francisco is contacted every week by wives of Anglican clergy who have just discovered their husbands have HIV infection and have been having sex with men. Personal communication.
52. Full discussion of hetersexual risks and uncertainties. *British Medical Journal*, 296 (1988): 1017–1020.
53. *Morbidity and Mortality* weekly report, 35 (1986): 76–79. See comments on page 31.
54. See Chapter 5 for non-sexual risks.
55. *Lancet*, 2 (1987): 40–41. Possibly a second case in *Annals of Internal Medicine*, 105: 6 (1986): 969.
56. *British Medical Journal*, 296 (1988): 1017–1020.
57. *Morbidity and Mortality Weekly Report*, 37: 3 (1988): 35–38.
58. *Christianity Today* (8 April 1988): 39.

Chapter 5 Questions People Ask

1. 'Female-to-Female Transmission of HIV,' *Lancet*, 2 (1987): 40–41.
2. *American Journal of Medicine*, 82: (1987): 188–189.
3. See pages 88, 89, and 116 for lists of preparations.
4. Further reading: 'AIDS – How You Catch It and How You Can't,' *New Scientist*, 113 (26 March 1987): 38–39.
5. Attempts are being made to develop a test for the virus that will detect HIV within days of infection. *Daily Express* (London: 11 November 1988).

6. *New Scientist*, 113 (26 March 1987): 37.
7. Ibid.
8. See page 69.
9. *American Journal of Public Health*, 78: 4 (1988): 462–467.
10. *New Scientist*, (19 February 1987): 58–59.
11. 'AIDS and the Condom—A Guide to Safer Sex,' London Rubber Company leaflet.
12. AIDS, 1: 1 (1987): 49–52.
13. *Independent* (19 December 1986).
14. *Journal of the American Medical Association, (JAMA)*, 255: 14 (1986): 1887–1891. One possible case of spread between footballers, *Lancet* 335 (1990) 1105.
15. Sports council for Wales lifted the ban in January 1987. *Guardian* (17 January 1987).
16. 'Stability and Inactivation of HTLV-III/LAV under Clinical and Laboratory Environments,' *Journal of the American Medical Association, (JAMA)*, 255: 14 (1986): 1887–1891.
17. *Lancet*, (1985): 188–189. Note: This paper suggests the virus is destroyed after 20 minutes' heating at fifty-six degrees, but they used an insensitive enzyme test (reverse transciptase).
18. 'Stability and Inactivation,' 1887–1891. See footnote 16.
19. Ibid.
20. Ibid.
21. *Journal of the American Medical Association*, 294 (1987): 1595–1597.
22. *Lancet*, 1 (1975): 188–189.
23. *British Medical Journal*, 294 (1987): 1595–1597.
24. *New York Times* (6 June 1987).
25. Safety guidelines: *British Dental Journal*, 162 (1987): 371–373, 375.
26. 'Design Improvements,' *New England Journal of Medicine* 319: 5 (1988): 284–288, 308.
27. British Medical Assocation, April 1990.
28. *Lancet*, 1 (1983): 925.
29. *Morbidity and Mortality* (22 May 1987): 285–288.
30. 'AIDS: A Doctor's Duty,' *British Medical Journal*, 294 (1987): 6. Also suggets a doctor might be struck off the register for refusing to look after someone with AIDS. The risk of getting hepatitis B infection is much greater than the risk of AIDS from a cut or scratch with a needle. *New England Journal of Medicine*, 312 (1985): 56–57.
31. Five million medical rubber gloves imported from Hong Kong to the United States had to be destroyed recently because they were full of holes. *Daily Telegraph* (8 November 1988).
32. *Lancet*, 2 (1986): 694. A second case was also reported.
33. Dr William Haseltine of Harvard Medical School was reported in the *New York Times* (18 March 1986) as saying that HIV could be transmitted

through mosquito bites.

34. 'No evidence for Arthropod Transmission of AIDS,' *Parasitology Today*, 2: 11 (1986): 294–295. One dissenting voice is a paper showing that in Africa poor housing and being near water courses made infection more likely, possibly due to insects.
35. *Bulletin of the World Health Association*, 65: 5 (1987): 607–613. There is no association with malaria except some extra cases of AIDS resulting directly from infected blood transfusions used to treat malaria anaemia. *Journal of the American Medical Association*, 259: 4 (1988): 545–549.
36. *Lancet*, 1 (1987): 1094–1098.
37. *Daily Telegraph* (London: 13 February 1987).
38. I must say that this conflicts with my own experience of serving on the other side of the altar rail in an Anglian church. I think the occasional fragment of a wafer is all I have ever seen.
39. Another vicar, the Rev Michael Moxon, Vicar of Tewkesbury Abbey, Gloucestershire, England, has been reported as telling his parishioners they need not drink the wine if they are afraid of infection by AIDS, *The Times* (5 January 1987).
40. Guidelines on AIDS and communion sent from Archbishops of Canterbury and York to all clergy in their pay slips (March 1987).
41. A hospital chaplain in Essex advised priests to wear rubber gloves and use a spatula when giving communion to people with AIDS! This is totally absurd (*The Times* [5 January 1987]). Medically trained people can be just as bad. In County Durham two ambulance personnel collected someone with AIDS in goggles and boiler suits (*Daily Mirror* [22 January 1987])! For a scientific discussion see *Journal of Infection*, 16: 1 (1988): 3–23.
42. *British Medical Journal*, 294 (1987): 433.
43. *Lancet*, 2 (1987): 132–133; 165–166. Proposes testing for new strains of HIV as well as old, in case some blood is missed.
44. National Blood Transfusion Service draft guidelines. Also 'The Patient's Blood Is the Safest Blood,' *New England Journal of Medicine*, 316: 9 (1987): 543–544; 'The Need for Autologous Blood Transfusions' *British Medical Journal*, 294 (1987): 307.
45. Longstanding practice in the United States (Florida): *Journal of the American Medical Association*, 257: 9 (1987): 1211–1214.
46. This occurred recently in Glasgow. A leukaemia patient was infected by a pint of blood which tested negative.
47. Many students were giving blood to get an HIV antibody test. *Daily Telegraph* report (London: 8 January 1987).
48. Transfusion centres were losing one hundred pints a day (15 per cent of their requirements). *The Times* (6 January 1987).
49. Haemophilia Society figures.
50. H. Jolly, *Diseases of Children* (Blackwell: 1981), 351.

51. *Morbidity and Mortality Weekly Report*, 36: 19 (1987): 285–288.
52. 'AIDS and First Aid,' *Occupational Health Review*, 6 (1987): 12.
53. *Journal of the American Medical Association*, 256: 22 (1986): 3092.
54. *Morbidity and Mortality Weekly Report*, 35: 45 (1986): 699–703; also *Morbidy and Mortality Weekly Report*, 36: 9 (1987): 133–135. TB is on the increase for the first time in decades, as more people develop AIDS.
55. *Tubercle*, 67: 4 (1986): 295–302.
56. *Quarterly Journal of Medicine*, 67: 254 (1988): 473–486.
57. A nurse and her husband have filed a lawsuit claiming $500 million against San Francisco General Hospital. They claim congenital defects in their baby were caused by cytomegalovirus picked up on the AIDS ward. *Mail on Sunday* (London: 14 February 1988): 15.
58. *British Medical Journal*, 295 (1987): 56.
59. *British Medical Journal*, 293 (1986): 489.
60. The British figures are partly explained by the absence of long-stay/hospice beds elsewhere. Demented patients in San Francisco General Hospital tend to go elsewhere. However, there is still a big difference.
61. *AIDSFILE*, 2 (1987): 2. San Francisco General Hospital Medical Centre; also *Chest* 88 (1985): 659–662; also *American Review of Respiratory Disease*, 133 (1986): 515–518.
62. 'Plotting the Spread of AIDS,' *New Scientist* (26 March 1986): 54–59.
63. *Reviews of Infectious Diseases*, 10:1 (1988): 138–150; 151–158.
64. *Journal of Sexually Transmitted Diseases*, 12 (1985): 203–208.
65. *Journal of Sexually Transmitted Diseases*, 12 (1985): 203–208.

Chapter 6 Condoms Are Unsafe

1. 'Cautions about Condoms in Prevention of AIDS,' *Lancet*, 1 (1987): 323.
2. Family Planning Association Leaflet. 'There Are Eight Methods of Birth Control' gives 3–15 per cent pregnant per year but the *Lancet* puts it at 13–15 per cent. *Lancet* 1 (1987): 323.
3. *Self Health* magazine survey, College of Health.
4. *Guardian* (21 July 1987). British Standard for imported brands. BSI for Durex is higher at one hole in two hundred condoms.
5. 'Can You Rely on Condoms?' *Consumer Reports* (March 1989): 136.
6. 'Cautions about Condoms,' 323. See footnote 1.
7. See endnote 2, this chapter.
8. Animated discussion with representative of Family Planning Association over this. Condom manufacuturers have to take this line for medico-legal reasons, otherwise they could be sued by a pregnant woman for making false claims—even more so now with AIDS.
9. *Medicine International*, (August 1988): 2332.

10. Terrence Higgins Trust literature advises: 'A condom should be used as a barrier in heterosexual lovemaking for both vaginal and anal sex. Do not rely on this as a method of birth control, *but use some other form of contraception to avoid pregnancy*.' 'Woman and AIDS,' 3.
11. An example: *Lancet*, 1(2/9 January 1988): 65.
12. *Journal of the American Medical Association*, (1987). Report showed only one in twelve became infected. Dangers of premature conclusions. In the brief interval between writing the paper and it being published, the number infected had already risen from one to three out of twelve. *New Scientist* (19 February 1987): 12.
13. *Scandinavian Journal of Infectious Diseases*, 20: 2 (1988): 233–234.
14. *New Scientist*, (26 February 1987): 61.
15. 'Women and AIDS.'
16. *The Times* (24 August 1987).
17. All condom instructions and AIDS prevention literature stress the importance of this.
18. *Lancet*, (1986): 527–529.
19. *Family Planning Today*, (2nd quarter, 1988): 1. Fifty per cent of the students said they would never use condoms—dulled sensitivity, broke, smelled, were embarrassing to use and meant sex had to be planned. Female condoms (eg. Femshield) are experimental but may be less disruptive—inserted by the woman, and reusable.
20. Forty-two per cent in recent survey of students. *The Times* (28 August 1987).
21. *British Medical Journal* 290 (1985): 1176.
22. Leisurewear marketeer Glenn's Style is giving away six condoms with every pair of jeans. *Marketing Weekly* (16 December 1988).
23. *Cosmopolitan* (January 1987).
24. *British Medical Journal*, 294 (1987): 1356.
25. See note 19.
26. *FIRSTAIDS ITV* (20 June 1987).
27. Recent opinion poll.
28. *Spermicides containing nonoxynol-9.*

    Delfen (cream or foam)
    Double Check (pessaries)
    Emko (foam)
    Gynol II (jelly)
    Ortho-cream (cream)
    Orthoforms (pessaries)
    Two's Company (pessaries)

    All these products are available from pharmacists or from your doctor. Brands of Durex containing spermicide contain nonoxynol-9, but only in small amounts.

29. Anxieties over pregnancy risks are lessened by recent reports. *Journal of the American Medical Association*, 261:9 (1989): 1289–1294.

Chapter 7 Moral Dilemmas

1. Voluntary Euthanasia Society opinion poll (1987) shows 30 per cent of family doctors in favour of legalisation – twice the 1985 figure. British Medical Association working party is reviewing recommendations.
2. Samaritans had record numbers of calls last year.
3. *AIDSFILE*, 2: 1 (1987): 6–7.
4. The fact that true depression always lifts has made it especially difficult to evaluate anti-depressant drugs, counselling, or anything else.
5. A terminal care team will usually provide patients, their friends and families, their doctors and nurses with a twenty-four-hour telephone number for help and advice.
6. Regular injections should now be a thing of the past with the new Graseby syringe driver. This is a large matchbox-sized, battery-operated device which holds a syringe containing all the medicines needed for twenty-four hours. The medicine drips in slowly under the skin through a minute needle and thin tube. Unlike big tubes in veins it is comfortable and can remain in place for a long time. These can be set up by a nurse at home or in hospital. Painkillers and sickness medicine are ideally given this way. However, many anti-AIDS drugs have to be given via a different route.
7. He has since died. He passed away peacefully with champagne on his lips a week later.
8. Medical Education Trust meeting in London (April 1987) came out strongly against euthanasia and advocated more widespread hospice care.
9. *New England Journal of Medicine*, 318: 15 (1988): 984–988.
10. As experience of doctors grows I hope many tests can be avoided. With any new disease the tendency is always to investigate first and consider options afterward. After a while common sense prevails and tests are done not to extend understanding of the disease, but only to enable correct treatment to be given. San Francisco now has excellent results in terms of patients' length of survival, with drastically fewer procedures. Hospital stays are greatly shortened (average eight days), and people spend much longer at home (see p. 103).
11. Up to thirty-six times more likely to commit suicide than general population. *Journal of the American Medical Association*, 259: 9 (1988): 1333–1337, sixty-six times in Cornell University study 1990.
12. A man: *Independent* (14 March 1987). A man—also shot wife and son;

and a woman—also killed husband and children: *The Times* (2 May 1987).

13. There is an antidote but it must be given within a few hours of taking the tablets. There has been some discussion about adding tiny doses of antidote to every tablet sold. It is suprising that such a lethal drug should be so widely available. The reason is that when the correct dose is taken, or higher doses are taken under medical supervision, it is one of the safest painkillers available. It also has virtually no side-effects such as drowsiness or constipation. Figures from Guy's Hospital Poison Centre.
14. Annual representative meeting of the British Medical Association (BMA) rejected World Health Organization and DHSS advice to pass the motion 'that testing for HIV antibody should be at the discretion of the patient's doctor, and should not necessarily require the consent of the patient.' BMA Chairman Dr John Marks has warned that patients could sue for assault (taking blood without consent) and doctors could be brought before the General Medical Council for discipline. It was also agreed that a result would not be passed on to other doctors without consent. New BMA and GMC guidelines available in *British Medical Journal*, 295 (1987): 73–74. The Medical Defence Union (MDU) says a doctor will not be prosecuted for informing a family doctor of a positive result without agreement from the patient so long as the family doctor needs the information to prevent the spread of disease or to treat the patient. *Journal of Medical Defense Union*, 2 (1986): 21–22.
15. Fraud: insurance companies are getting scared. They think there have been several cases where someone has known he is positive, or been almost certain, and has taken out a massive life insurance policy. The family doctor, of course, for reasons discussed earlier is totally unaware of the diagnosis—often even if his patient has full-blown AIDS. The insurance company gets a letter saying the patient is fit and has not been having medical treatment for any condition and issues the policy. Several instances are being investigated. In one case the company was convinced that $630,000 paid to the homosexual lover was for a man who died of AIDS and that it was the result of false information on the original policy. However, because the hospital refused to give any information and the death certificate said 'pneumonia'—as it usually does—nothing could be checked. Scottish Equitable now insists on blood tests and Standard Life Assurance is refusing cover in most cases where two men are jointly purchasing property (*Sunday Express* [25 January 1987]; also *Financial Times* [30 January 1987]). California and Washington, DC, have already made it illegal for insurers to use HIV antibody tests. BUPA and Private Patients Plan have paid for private medical care for a few people with AIDS but only where they were certain the policy started before infection was known (*Today* [13 January 1987]). In the future, BUPA will not pay for AIDS care where the person has been insured for less than five

years, and Private Patients Plan will only pay for initial diagnosis and treatment. *Sunday Telegraph* (5 July 1987).

16. *Canadian Medical Association Journal*, 139: 15 (1988): 287–288; also *New England Journal of Medicine*, 319: 15 (1988): 1010–1012. Articles outline the debate in greater detail.
17. A survey showed many hospital consultants were confused over the legal requirements and options. *Lancet*, 1 (1987): 26–28.
18. A gay doctor writes that he would inform a hospital if admitted for an operation that he could have AIDS, but would expect the surgeon to be fired if he refused to operate (*British Medical Journal*, 294 [1987]: 647). See also glossary (p. 235) for description of sex change operations and some issues invovled. Ethical code for physicians regarding treatment of people with AIDS: *Journal of the American Medical Association*, 259: 4 (1988): 1360–1361.
19. 'AIDS: A Bill of Rights for the Surgical Team,' *British Medical Journal*, 296 (1988): 490.
20. *Canadian Medical Association Journal*, 138: 6 (1988): 490.
21. TV news bulletin (June 1987).
22. A large United States study concluded that only a third of such accidents were preventable (*New England Journal of Medicine*, 314 [1986]: 1127–1132). If minor, each accident may only transmit infection in one out of two hundred cases, but the catalogue of accidents is going to become enormous as the number of people needing treatment for AIDS continues to rise rapidly.
23. *Guardian* (5 January 1987). Report on BBC fourteen-point plan to prevent spread of AIDS. A laboratory worker at the Royal Hallamshire Hospital in Sheffield was suspended after refusing to handle blood samples he thought could be infected. *The Times* (24 December 1986).
24. AIDS risk for NHS staff greater outside work. *Health and Safety Journal*, 97 (1987): 33.
25. Ealing Health Authority guidelines ICP23 (November 1986) for operating theatres: 'Ideally the theatre should be allowed to "rest" for at least twelve hours following the operation'—allows fine aerosol mists to settle. 'Student nurses and medical students should be excluded ... After the operation the theatre should be thoroughly cleaned with hot water and detergent. All surfaces should be wiped with detergent hypochlorate.' Similar rules exist for X-ray departments. Some argue that testing does not rule out infection completely. True, but it picks up the majority—after all, testing blood is worthwhile and very few infected donations are missed.
26. *British Medical Journal*, 294 (1987): 44.
27. *Journal of Occupational Medicine*, 30:7 (1988): 578–579: AIDS guidelines for occupational physicians. Employers who breach confidentiality may face charges of invasion of privacy, defamation and inten-

tional infliction of emotional distress with heavy fines. *Occupational Health and Safety*, 57: 7 (1988): 12–19; 31.

28. Sir Richard Doll, chairman of epidemiological subcommittee of Medical Research Council's AIDS working party argued strongly in favour. *British Medical Journal*, 294 (1987): 244.
29. *The Times* (16 November 1988).
30. *International Herald Tribune* (2 February 1988): 4.
31. *Today* (4 February 1987).
32. This is legal by Act of Parliament—Public Health (Control of Disease) Act (1984) and Public Health (Infectious Disease) regulations (1985).
33. *The Times* (21 March 1987).
34. *The Times* (23 March 1987).
35. *Law Society Gazette* (25 March 1987). It is now a crime for a doctor not to inform a spouse in some parts of the United States.
36. *New England Journal of Medicine*, 316: 16 (1987): 1924.
37. Two lawyers have suggested liability to prosecution under the British Offences Against the Persons Act of 1861 for 'maliciously administering any poison or other destructive and noxious thing.'
38. *Independent* (21 August 1987).
39. *Sunday Express* (11 January 1987).
40. *Sunday Express* (7 June 1987).
41. *AIDS-Forschung*, 2: 11 (1987): 648–651. Munich court judgement.
42. *British Journal of Hospital Medicine*; also *The Times* (15 July 1987). Many prostitutes insist on clients using condoms but often a two tier pricing system exists—if you want it without, you pay more. *Health Education Journal*, 46: 2 (August 1987): 71–73.
43. 'Identity Cards for People Infected with HIV?', *British Medical Journal*, 294 (1987): 772.
44. *Lancet*, 1 (1987): 982–983. Reports twenty-one instances in one London clinic alone.
45. 'Summary of AIDS Law Worldwide,' *AIDS-Forschung*, 1: 9 (1986): 505–513.

Chapter 8 Wrath or Reaping?

1. 'Because of this, God gave them over to shameful lusts. Even their women exchanged natural relations with women and were inflamed with lust for one another. Men committed indecent acts with men and received in themselves the due penalty for their perversion' (Rom. 1:26–27).
2. One of the latest of these pronouncements from the Church Society is 'AIDS and the Judgement of God' (July 1987). It states, 'Twice in the

AIDS debate, in two separate evangelical publications, it has been written that God does not "zap" individuals. The Bible witness is that he sometimes does.' The report stresses the 'sinful nature of homosexual practices' and that God does judge 'here and now'. The United States Bishops of the United Methodist Church disagree—God does not 'wage germ warfare on the human family.' *International Herald Tribune* (9 May 1988).

3. The exact words recorded in Greek are 'Let the sinless one cast the first stone.' Translated in the New International Version of the Bible as: 'If any one of you is without sin, let him be the first to throw a stone at her.' You can read this story in John 8.1–11.
4. Literally, 'From now, no longer sin' (John 8:11, New English Bible).
5. "You have heard that it was said to the people long ago, 'Do not commit adultery.' But I tell you that anyone who looks at a woman lustfully has already committed adultery with her in his heart" (Matt. 5:27–28).
6. "You have heard that it was said to the people long ago, 'Do not murder, and anyone who murders will be subject to judgment.' But I tell you that anyone who is angry with his brother will be subject to judgment' (Matt. 5:21–22).
7. "For the words that the mouth utters come from the overflowing of the heart" (Matt. 12:34, New English Bible). This is not to say that all wrongdong is treated the same by God: Scripture shows clearly that some actions and attitudes particularly invoke his anger. We are not looking here at God's reactions in his holy judgement, but at the right of mortal, imperfect humans to stand on a pedestal and condemn others.
8. 'For all have sinned and fall short of the glory of God' (Rom. 3:23).
9. 'Because he himself suffered when he was tempted, he is able to help those who are being tempted' (Heb. 2:18).
10. Personal communcations from National Childwatch.
11. National Childwatch 60 Beck Rd., Everthorpe, South Care, Brough, E. Yorks.
12. 'But you are a chosen people, a royal priesthood, a holy nation, a people belonging to God, that you may declare the praises of him who called you out of darkness into his wonderful light' (1 Pet. 2:9).
13. 'I urge you to live a life worthy of the calling you have received' (Eph. 4:1).
14. 1 Timothy 3:2–15. The one exception in the list is being 'able to teach.'
15. 'Jesus answered them: "It is not the healthy who need a doctor, but the sick. I have not come to call the righteous, but sinners to repentance."' (Luke 5:31–32).
16. Luke 23:43. God's forgiveness when we are truly sorry is absolute.
17. Genesis 12–23.
18. Genesis 2:24; Matthew 19:4–6; 1 Corinthians 6:16.
19. There are those who quote from the Bible (e.g., Romans 1:26–27) to

argue that certain sexual sins are particularly abhorrent to God. (See page 135 of this chapter.) The day we start ranking our own or others' sins in some kind of scale of sinfulness is the day we attempt to make God's grace null and void. 'I only lied, cheated, and stole—I didn't commit buggery. I am a reasonably good-natured sort of person—I *deserve* to go to heaven.' The Bible teaches that separation is separation. Even the most humanly perfect person is so imperfect as to be impossibly separated. The only exception is Jesus. You need to read the story again about the woman caught in adultery. There was no such grading in Jesus' mind when he rebuked the crowd. Read the rest of Romans 1: the rest of the list includes gossip and jealousy—but we ignore these. The vital phrase, 'giving them over', is used in verses 24, 26, and 28—not just of sexual sin. The basis of God's anger is explained in verse 21: 'They know God, but do not give him the honour that belongs to him' (Good News Bible).

20. John 14:6. Also see Acts 4:12.
21. 'For it is by grace you have been saved, through faith—and this not from yourselves, it is the gift of God—not by works, so that no one can boast' (Eph. 2:8–9).
22. 'Therefore, if anyone is in Christ, he is a new creation; the old has gone, the new has come!' (2 Cor. 5:17).
23. John 3:3.
24. Romans 6:8.
25. Romans 6:3–4.
26. Galatians 2:20, New English Bible.
27. No. They weren't amazed because he'd cut his hair and started wearing a suit. His appearance was exactly the same but something *inside* had changed. The church is so good at sucking people in and pushing identical people out at the other end: same jokes, same dress, same mannerisms. The Christian ghetto rules. The day that happens in my church I want out!
28. Romans 7:14–25. For discussion of Holy Spirit, see page 159.
29. 1 Corinthians 10:13; Philippians 4:13.
30. John 4:4–30.
31. Luke 19:45; Matthew 21:12–13; Mark 11:15–16.
32. Greek word used is *Ek-ballo*—literally to 'throw out'.
33. Luke 10:25–37.
34. 'You have heard that it was said, "Love your neighbour and hate your enemy." But I tell you, love your enemies and pray for those who persecute you, that you may be sons of your Father in heaven' (Matt. 5:43–45).
35. 'He is patient with you, not wanting anyone to perish, but everyone to come to repentance' (2 Pet. 3:9).
36. Acts 4:12. Separation is the consequence of going our own way and is, I believe, the so-called penalty mentioned in Romans 1:26–27.

37. 'This will happen when the Lord Jesus is revealed from heaven in blazing fire with his powerful angels. He will punish those who do not know God and do not obey the gospel of our Lord Jesus. They will be punished with everlasting destruction and shut out from the presence of the Lord and from the majesty of his power on the day he comes to be glorified in his holy people and to be marvelled at among all those who have believed' (2 Thess. 1:7–10).
38. Galatians 6:7.
39. Ephesians 1:10.
40. 2 Peter 3:9.
41. Matthew 12:36.
42. Luke 9:24, New English Bible.
43. Mark 9:47, New English Bible.
44. John 1:12, Romans 8:14–17.
45. 'But among you there must not be even a hint of sexual immorality, or of any kind of impurity, or of greed, because these are improper for God's holy people' (Eph. 5:3–5).
46. 1 Corinthians 7:32–37.
47. This is a large but incomplete list. The reason I have given it is that many people have never really understood what the Bible says on these subjects.

    (a) Adultery: Exodus 20:14; Leviticus 20:10; Job 24:15; Matthew 5:27; 19:9; Romans 7:3; 1 Corinthians 6:9; 2 Peter 2:14.

    (b) Sex outside marriage (general references): Matthew 5:28; Romans 1:24; 6:19; Ephesians 4:19; 5:3; Colossians 3:5; 1 Thessalonians 4:7; Hebrews 13:4; 2 Peter 2:10. *Specific references:* Matthew 5:32; Acts 15:29; 1 Corinthians 5:1; 6:18; 7:2; 10:8; 1 Thessalonians 4:3.

    (c) Bad attitudes (Lust): Proverbs 6:25; Matthew 5:28; Galatians 5:16; Colossians 3:5; 1 Thessalonians 4:5; 2 Timothy 2:22; James 1:15; 1 Peter 2:11.

    (d) Homosexual practices as a type of sex outside marriage: Genesis 19; Leviticus 18:22; 20:13; Judges 19:22; Romans 1:27; 1 Corinthians 6:9; 1 Timothy 1:10; 2 Peter 2:4–10; Jude 7.
48. Ephesians 4:26.
49. Ephesians 5:18.
50. 1 Corinthians 13.
51. 'If we say that we have no sin, we are only fooling ourselves, and refusing to accept the truth. But if we confess our sins to him, he can be depended on to forgive us and to cleanse us from every wrong' (1 John 1:8–9, The Living Bible).

Chapter 9 Life and Death Issues

1. Imagine the fuss if I had been taking pictures of what happens in a crematorium—of what really happens on the other side of the curtain.
2. Philippians 3;8–14.
3. Philippians 1:27.
4. For example, John Wimber's *Power Healing* (Hodder and Stoughton, 1986). A surprisingly balanced book on exercising the gift of healing. Wimber has had an enormous influence on churches as part of the so-called 'charismatic renewal' with its emphasis on God working here and now in supernatural ways. Many rapidly-growing churches have a strong charismatic influence, regardless of their denominational labels.
5. Elizabeth Burnham, *When Your Friend Is Dying* (Kingsway, 1982) is a first-hand account of being on the receiving end.
6. Cadaveric instrumentation is widely practised. The argument is that the patient has died and practising the technique could save a life. The veins usually used for injections empty of blood when the heart stops so are hard to find. Occasionally the only way to inject a drug to try and start the heart again is into a vein deep inside the body. Getting a needle in the right place can be hard. Here is my personal view:
(a) If the patient is dead, then ethically it is not right to experiment without permission of next of kin.
(b) If, as I believe, the patient is usually still dying, then I should act according to what I think the patient would prefer.
(c) The technique is usually practised furtively, in haste, behind closed curtains, with an eye over the shoulder in case relatives arrive. This is not ethical behaviour.
(d) The test is this: Would you ever be able to confess to relatives that you had carried on jabbing, etc., for practice, or would they be too distressed at the thought?
(e) Instrumentation in this way distracts the team from changing gear. It prevents a peaceful death. It robs the patient of a last moment or two of dignity. It delays the introduction of a spouse to the dying patient.
(f) If no relatives or close friends are present outside, I think it permissible for the junior doctor concerned to *ask* any other team member remaining if he or she minds. If permission is granted then one or two brief attempts only and then call it a day. Intubation is easily practised in medical school seven days a week. Subclavian cannulation (inserting a plastic tube into a vein under the shoulder blade to administer drugs during cardiac arrest) is not such a tremendous technique in an arrest. In most cases it will not affect the outcome. I do not think it necessary for every junior in a big hospital to practise this on corpses. Doctors would do *far* better to *practise heart massage*. A recent study showed that the vast majority of fully qualified hospital doctors could not even massage

the heart adequately enough to prevent brain damage (Royal College of Physicians: 'Resuscitation from Cardiopulmonary Arrest.' Training and Organisation. Report July 1987). No wonder so many attempts result in failure: too many doctors being too clever with too many fancy drugs and needles. Yet this is another example of an appalling lack of common sense in medicine.

We should stand for the rights of the patient, and should show our colleagues that the moments of dying are hallowed ground.

7. Luke 23:40–43.
8. Matthew 19:30; 20:16; Mark 9:35; Luke 13:30.

Chapter 10 A Plan for the Government

1. Ugandan results were 800,000 estimated infected (1988).
2. *Toronto Star* (17 February 1989).
3. Conservative estimate is $80,000 per patient (*Science USA*, 239 [5 February 1988]: 604–610). Some argue that there are no hospital costs: the bed is there anyway; all that happens is that it is filled by someone with AIDS rather than someone with heart disease. Early on when numbers of people with AIDS are small that may be true, but we are already at the stage of planning extra beds which otherwise would not have existed or would have been closed, as a result of AIDS, and the epidemic's effects have hardly begun.
4. Twelve million dollars in federal funds has established thirteen Regional Education and Training Centres to train health care providers. *Journal of the American Medical Association*, 260: 4 (1988): 2016; also *Morbidity and Mortality Weekly Report* (guidelines for schools), 37: S2 (1988).
5. *Pediatrics*, 82:2 (1988): 278–280 (American Academy of Pediatrics Committee on School Health).
6. This has always been so for courses on other subjects before AIDS. A Bradford conference for family doctors on AIDS was attended by only ten. *The Times* (24 April 1987).
7. *New York Times* (22 September 1987). Reported fifty-eight homeless in New York hospitals with AIDS. Most needed practical help at home or nursing care. Shortages exist in the community of places and of caseworkers to help place people.
8. Personal communication.

Chapter 11 A Strategy for the Church

1. Hospice of St Martin, Florida, annual report (1987–1988).

Chapter 12 What You Can Do about AIDS

1. *AIDS-Forschung*, 3:7 (1988): 392–401; also *Journal of the American Medical Association*, 258: 14 (1987): 1969.
2. *Holistic Medicine*, 2: 4 (1987): 203–215.

Appendix B Burnout Among AIDS Care Workers—How to Spot It, How to Avoid It

1. Term first introduced by Freudenberger in 1974. *Journal of Social Issues*, 30 (1984): 159–165; *British Medical Journal*, 295 (1987): 284–285.
2. John 11:35.
3. See 'Withholding treatment,' p. 123.

Appendix C Advice to Travellers Going Abroad

1. *Lancet*, 2 (13 August, 1988): 394–395.

Appendix D Checklist of Countries

1. Figures obtained from the World Health Organization and Centre for Disease Control. (1 March 1989). Excellent article on world situation, *Scientific American* (October 1988): 60–69.
2. World Health Organisation firgures, *New England Journal of Medicine*, 319; 5 (1988): 302–303.
3. *The Times* (28 August 1987).
4. *New Scientist*, 7 (January 1988): 36–37.
5. Panos Institute (1987).
6. Pattern II is observed in areas of central, eastern, and southern Africa and in some Caribbean countries. In these countries, most of the reported cases occur in heterosexuals; the male-to-female ratio is approximately 1:1; and perinatal transmission is more common than in other areas. Intravenous drug use and homosexual transmission either do not occur or occur at a low level.
7. Includes 1 tissue recipient and 8 transfusion recipients who received blood screened for HIV antibody.
8. 'Other' is 2 heath-care workers who seroconverted to HIV and developed AIDS after occupational exposure to HIV-infected blood. 'Undertermined' refers to patients who died, were lost to follow-up, or

refused interview; and those whose mode of exposure to HIV remains undetermined after investigation.

9. Pattern II is observed in areas of central, eastern, and southern Africa and in some Caribbean countires. In these countries, most of the reported cases occur in heterosexuals; the male-to-female ratio is approximately 1:1; and perinatal transmission is more common than in other areas. Intravenous drug use and homosexual transmission either do not occur or occur at a low level.

Index

Aids And Young People

by Dr Patrick Dixon

With each year that passes more and more people know someone with AIDS. People with AIDS are often young and illness is not their only problem...Prospects of housing, employment, insurance and even friendship can change rapidly.

—If you've lost a friend, or fear that you may do soon
—If you're still unsure about what AIDS can do

then this book will speak to you in a direct and no-nonsense way.

PATRICK DIXON is a doctor and church leader with many years' experience of caring for the dying. He is the Director of ACET—AIDS Care Education and Training—and author of the highly acclaimed book The Truth About AIDS.

Kingsway Publications

Kingsway Publications

Kingsway Publications publishes books to encourage spiritual values in the home, church and society. The list includes Bibles, popular paperbacks, more specialist volumes, booklets, and a range of children's fiction.

Kingsway Publications is owned by The Servant Trust, a Christian charity run by representatives of the evangelical church in Britain, committed to serve God in publishing and music.

For further information on the Trust, including details of how you may be able to support its work, please write to:

The Secretary
The Servant Trust
1 St Anne's Road
Eastbourne
East Sussex BN21 3UN
England